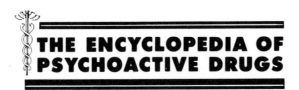

THE ENCYCLOPEDIA OF PSYCHOACTIVE DRUGS

SERIES 1

SERIES 2

DRUGS
&
THE ARTS

GENERAL EDITOR
Professor Solomon H. Snyder, M.D.
*Distinguished Service Professor of
Neuroscience, Pharmacology, and Psychiatry at
The Johns Hopkins University School of Medicine*

•

ASSOCIATE EDITOR
Professor Barry L. Jacobs, Ph.D.
*Program in Neuroscience, Department of Psychology,
Princeton University*

•

SENIOR EDITORIAL CONSULTANT
Joann Rodgers
*Deputy Director, Office of Public Affairs at
The Johns Hopkins Medical Institutions*

SOLOMON H. SNYDER, M.D. • GENERAL EDITOR

THE ENCYCLOPEDIA OF PSYCHOACTIVE DRUGS

SERIES 2

DRUGS & THE ARTS

MARC KUSINITZ

CHELSEA HOUSE PUBLISHERS

NEW YORK • NEW HAVEN • PHILADELPHIA

EDITOR-IN-CHIEF: Nancy Toff
EXECUTIVE EDITOR: Remmel T. Nunn
MANAGING EDITOR: Karyn Gullen Browne
COPY CHIEF: Perry Scott King
ART DIRECTOR: Giannella Garrett
PICTURE EDITOR: Elizabeth Terhune

STAFF FOR DRUGS AND THE ARTS:

SENIOR EDITOR: Jane Larkin Crain
ASSOCIATE EDITOR: Paula Edelson
ASSISTANT EDITOR: Michele A. Merens
DESIGNER: Victoria Tomaselli
COPY EDITORS: Sean Dolan, Gillian Bucky
CAPTIONS: Louise Bloomfield
PICTURE RESEARCH: Diane Moroff
PRODUCTION COORDINATOR: Alma Rodriguez

CREATIVE DIRECTOR: Harold Steinberg

COVER: Joseph Ciardiello

Library of Congress Cataloging-in-Publication Data
Kusinitz, Marc.
   Drugs & the arts.
   (The encyclopedia of psychoactive drugs. Series 2)
   Bibliography: p.
   Includes index.
   Summary: Examines the impact drugs have made among
creative professionals in dance, art, music, theatre, and
motion pictures and discusses artistic works that portray the
world of drugs and drug abuse.
   1. Drugs and the arts—Juvenile literature. 2. Artists—Drug
use—History—Juvenile literature. 3. Drug abuse—History—
Juvenile literature. [1. Drugs and the arts. 2. Artists—Drug
use. 3. Drug abuse—History] I. Title. II. Title: Drugs and the
arts. III. Series.
NX180.D78K87   1987   700'.1'03   87-5179

ISBN 1-55546-224-3

CONTENTS

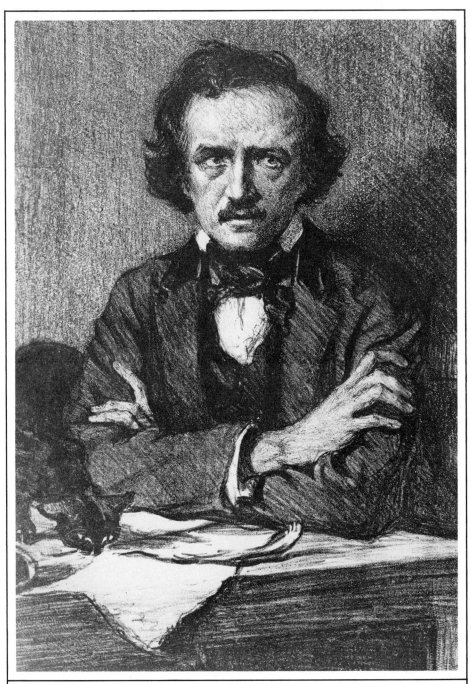

19th-century American author Edgar Allan Poe is best known for his classically macabre stories. Like many artists before and since, Poe wove drug-induced visions into his tales of horror and the grotesque.

In the Mainstream of American Life

One of the legacies of the social upheaval of the 1960s is that psychoactive drugs have become part of the mainstream of American life. Schools, homes, and communities cannot be "drug proofed." There is a demand for drugs — and the supply is plentiful. Social norms have changed and drugs are not only available—they are everywhere.

But where efforts to curtail the supply of drugs and outlaw their use have had tragically limited effects on demand, it may be that education has begun to stem the rising tide of drug abuse among young people and adults alike.

Over the past 25 years, as drugs have become an increasingly routine facet of contemporary life, a great many teenagers have adopted the notion that drug taking was somehow a right or a privilege or a necessity. They have done so, however, without understanding the consequences of drug use during the crucial years of adolescence.

The teenage years are few in the total life cycle, but critical in the maturation process. During these years adolescents face the difficult tasks of discovering their identity, clarifying their sexual roles, asserting their independence, learning to cope with authority, and searching for goals that will give their lives meaning.

Drugs rob adolescents of precious time, stamina, and health. They interrupt critical learning processes, sometimes forever. Teenagers who use drugs are likely to withdraw increasingly into themselves, to "cop out" at just the time when they most need to reach out and experience the world.

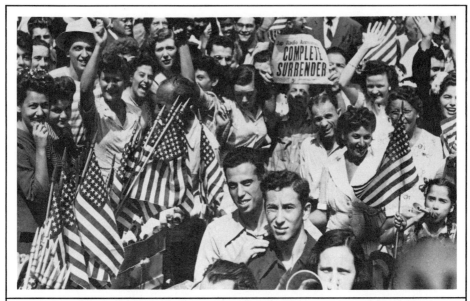

Crowds celebrate the end of World War II. The postwar era ushered in a time of unprecedented prosperity in America, but it also spawned the Beat movement, led by a group of artists who rejected material values and used drugs to demonstrate their alienation from mainstream society.

Fortunately, as a recent Gallup poll shows, young people are beginning to realize this, too. They themselves label drugs their most important problem. In the last few years, moreover, the climate of tolerance and ignorance surrounding drugs has been changing.

Adolescents as well as adults are becoming aware of mounting evidence that every race, ethnic group, and class is vulnerable to drug dependency.

Recent publicity about the cost and failure of drug rehabilitation efforts; dangerous drug use among pilots, air traffic controllers, star athletes, and Hollywood celebrities; and drug-related accidents, suicides, and violent crime have focused the public's attention on the need to wage an all-out war on drug abuse before it seriously undermines the fabric of society itself.

The anti-drug message is getting stronger and there is evidence that the message is beginning to get through to adults and teenagers alike.

The Encyclopedia of Psychoactive Drugs hopes to play a part in the national campaign now underway to educate young people about drugs. Series 1 provides clear and comprehensive discussions of common psychoactive substances, outlines their psychological and physiological effects on the mind and body, explains how they "hook" the user, and separates fact from myth in the complex issue of drug abuse.

Whereas Series 1 focuses on specific drugs, such as nicotine or cocaine, Series 2 confronts a broad range of both social and physiological phenomena. Each volume addresses the ramifications of drug use and abuse on some aspect of human experience: social, familial, cultural, historical, and physical. Separate volumes explore questions about the effects of drugs on brain chemistry and unborn children; the use and abuse of painkillers; the relationship between drugs and sexual behavior, sports, and the arts; drugs and disease; the role of drugs in history; and the sophisticated drugs now being developed in the laboratory that will profoundly change the future.

Each book in the series is fully illustrated and is tailored to the needs and interests of young readers. The more adolescents know about drugs and their role in society, the less likely they are to misuse them.

Joann Rodgers
Senior Editorial Consultant

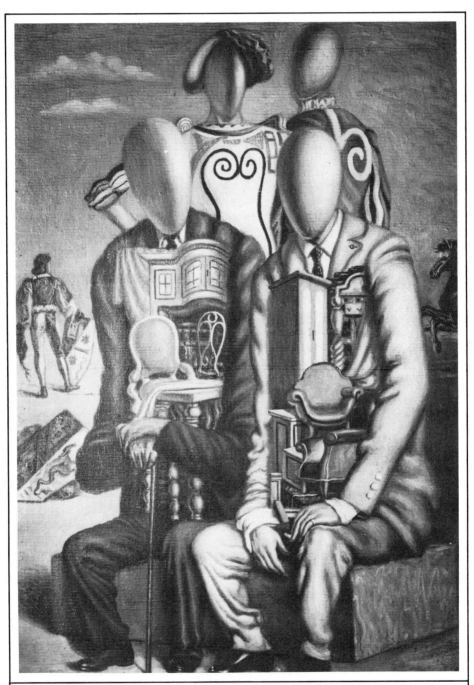

Gentleman in Borghese, *by Giorgio de Chirico. The juxtaposition of realism and nightmare is typical of surrealist painting. Many artists used similar images in an attempt to transcend everyday reality.*

The Gift of Wizardry
Use and Abuse

JACK H. MENDELSON, M.D.
NANCY K. MELLO, Ph.D.

Alcohol and Drug Abuse Research Center
Harvard Medical School—McLean Hospital

Dorothy to the Wizard:

"I think you are a very bad man," said Dorothy.
"Oh no, my dear; I'm really a very good man; but I'm a very bad Wizard."
—from THE WIZARD OF OZ

Man is endowed with the gift of wizardry, a talent for discovery and invention. The discovery and invention of substances that change the way we feel and behave are among man's special accomplishments, and, like so many other products of our wizardry, these substances have the capacity to harm as well as to help. Psychoactive drugs can cause profound changes in the chemistry of the brain and other vital organs, and although their legitimate use can relieve pain and cure disease, their abuse leads in a tragic number of cases to destruction.

Consider alcohol — available to all and yet regarded with intense ambivalence from biblical times to the present day. The use of alcoholic beverages dates back to our earliest ancestors. Alcohol use and misuse became associated with the worship of gods and demons. One of the most powerful Greek gods was Dionysus, lord of fruitfulness and god of wine. The Romans adopted Dionysus but changed his name to Bacchus. Festivals and holidays associated with Bacchus celebrated the harvest and the origins of life. Time has blurred the images of the Bacchanalian festival, but the theme of drunkenness as a major part of celebration has survived the pagan gods and remains a familiar part of modern society. The term "Bacchanalian Festival" conveys a more appealing image than "drunken orgy" or "pot party," but whatever the label, drinking alcohol is a form of drug use that results in addiction for millions.

The fact that many millions of other people can use alcohol in moderation does not mitigate the toll this drug takes on society as a whole. According to reliable estimates, one out of every ten Americans develops a serious alcohol-related problem sometime in his or her lifetime. In addition, automobile accidents caused by drunken drivers claim the lives of tens of thousands every year. Many of the victims are gifted young people, just starting out in adult life. Hospital emergency rooms abound with patients seeking help for alcohol-related injuries.

Who is to blame? Can we blame the many manufacturers who produce such an amazing variety of alcoholic beverages? Should we blame the educators who fail to explain the perils of intoxication, or so exaggerate the dangers of drinking that no one could possibly believe them? Are friends to blame — those peers who urge others to "drink more and faster," or the macho types who stress the importance of being able to "hold your liquor"? Casting blame, however, is hardly constructive, and pointing the finger is a fruitless way to deal with the problem. Alcoholism and drug abuse have few culprits but many victims. Accountability begins with each of us, every time we choose to use or misuse an intoxicating substance.

It is ironic that some of man's earliest medicines, derived from natural plant products, are used today to poison and to intoxicate. Relief from pain and suffering is one of society's many continuing goals. Over 3,000 years ago, the Therapeutic Papyrus of Thebes, one of our earliest written records, gave instructions for the use of opium in the treatment of pain. Opium, in the form of its major derivative, morphine, and similar compounds, such as heroin, have also been used by many to induce changes in mood and feeling. Another example of man's misuse of a natural substance is the coca leaf, which for centuries was used by the Indians of Peru to reduce fatigue and hunger. Its modern derivative, cocaine, has important medical use as a local anesthetic. Unfortunately, its increasing abuse in the 1980s clearly has reached epidemic proportions.

The purpose of this series is to explore in depth the psychological and behavioral effects that psychoactive drugs have on the individual, and also, to investigate the ways in which drug use influences the legal, economic, cultural, and even moral aspects of societies. The information presented here (and in other books in this series) is based on many clinical and laboratory studies and other observations by people from diverse walks of life.

Over the centuries, novelists, poets, and dramatists have provided us with many insights into the sometimes seductive but ultimately problematic aspects of alcohol and drug use. Physicians, lawyers, biologists, psychologists, and social scientists have contributed to a better understanding of the causes and consequences of using these substances. The authors in this series have attempted to gather and condense all the latest information about drug use and abuse. They have also described the sometimes wide gaps in our knowledge and have suggested some new ways to answer many difficult questions.

One such question, for example, is how do alcohol and drug problems get started? And what is the best way to treat them when they do? Not too many years ago, alcoholics and drug abusers were regarded as evil, immoral, or both. It is now recognized that these persons suffer from very complicated diseases involving deep psychological and social problems. To understand how the disease begins and progresses, it is necessary to understand the nature of the substance, the behavior of addicts, and the characteristics of the society or culture in which they live.

Although many of the social environments we live in are very similar, some of the most subtle differences can strongly influence our thinking and behavior. Where we live, go to school and work, whom we discuss things with — all influence our opinions about drug use and misuse. Yet we also share certain commonly accepted beliefs that outweigh any differences in our attitudes. The authors in this series have tried to identify and discuss the central, most crucial issues concerning drug use and misuse.

Despite the increasing sophistication of the chemical substances we create in the laboratory, we have a long way to go in our efforts to make these powerful drugs work for us rather than against us.

The volumes in this series address a wide range of timely questions. What influence has drug use had on the arts? Why do so many of today's celebrities and star athletes use drugs, and what is being done to solve this problem? What is the relationship between drugs and crime? What is the physiological basis for the power drugs can hold over us? These are but a few of the issues explored in this far-ranging series.

Educating people about the dangers of drugs can go a long way towards minimizing the desperate consequences of substance abuse for individuals and society as a whole. Luckily, human beings have the resources to solve even the most serious problems that beset them, once they make the commitment to do so. As one keen and sensitive observer, Dr. Lewis Thomas, has said,

> There is nothing at all absurd about the human condition. We matter. It seems to me a good guess, hazarded by a good many people who have thought about it, that we may be engaged in the formation of something like a mind for the life of this planet. If this is so, we are still at the most primitive stage, still fumbling with language and thinking, but infinitely capacitated for the future. Looked at this way, it is remarkable that we've come as far as we have in so short a period, really no time at all as geologists measure time. We are the newest, youngest, and the brightest thing around.

DRUGS
&
THE ARTS

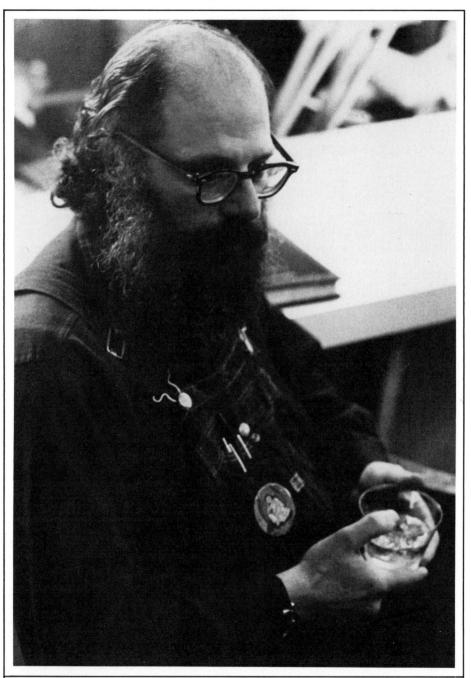

Allen Ginsberg, a prominent member of America's Beat movement. Like some of their artistic forebears, many of the Beats experimented with drugs and recorded their experiences in prose and poetry.

AUTHOR'S PREFACE

Throughout much of the world, the drug abuse problem affects all aspects of society. Schoolchildren, corporate executives, sports stars, physicians, and construction workers, as well as inner-city residents filled with despair and disappointment, are all among the ranks of drug abusers and addicts.

The artistic community is part of society, and so it should be no surprise that it too has members who abuse drugs. The history of drug use by artists, in fact, is much longer than that of most, if not all, other segments of society in the United States and other countries.

Artists have traditionally looked to new experiences to help them understand or express their creative urges. The use of psychoactive substances is just one of those experiences. Unfortunately, these substances work because they affect the brain — the very tool that makes an artist more than just a pair of moving hands or a set of vibrating vocal cords.

Thus, despite the important role that life experiences play in the arts, drugs have often destroyed the talents — and the lives — of artists who used them. What starts out as a shortcut to the creative impulse ends as a short circuit of the artistic current within the drug user. Nevertheless, the lure of drugs, with their promise of mind-expanding experiences and soothing relief from painful realities, continues to seduce artists.

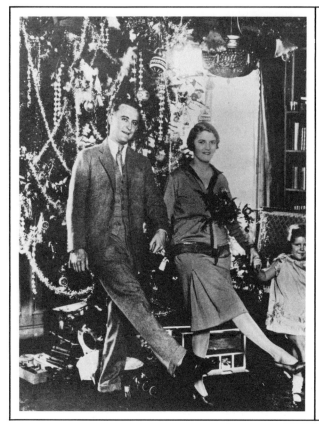

F. Scott Fitzgerald and his wife, Zelda, in 1925. Fitzgerald, whose novels describe the trendy but jaded high society of the jazz age, was himself a victim of the era's perils. After years of heavy drinking, he died of alcoholism in 1940.

    Drugs and the Arts is a survey of the influence of psychoactive drugs on the artistic community. Although this volume covers many hundreds of years of history, it is not comprehensive and is not intended to be. Rather, this book is an introduction to the topic of how drugs have affected art and artists throughout history. It is in some ways a social history, too, as well as an examination of how artists of one generation have influenced those of another.

    Chapter 1 examines the earliest references to drugs in ancient Asian and European tales and legends. It also surveys representations of psychoactive substances in world literature from those times through the early 19th century. Chapter 2 discusses the literary influences of different drugs on particular artistic movements. Chapter 3 explores the impact of drugs on the pioneers and performers of a truly American art form — jazz. Returning to the literary world, Chapter 4 discusses the effects of psychoactive drugs on the works and lives of some 20th-century authors. Chapter 5 examines the attitudes of different 20th-century plays and movies toward the use of drugs. Chapter 6 discusses the connection between drugs and the age-old art form of dance. Finally, Chapter 7 explores how the myths and realities of psychoactive drugs have influenced the work of a wide range of both Western and Eastern painters and sculptors.

It is important to note that the question of whether drugs are necessary, or even useful, to the creative process is not answered definitively here. What is clearly demonstrated, however, is the destructive potential of drugs to the artistic process, as well as individual examples of how drug abuse has affected particular artists. Although this might seem like moralizing, it is an inescapable lesson. It is a lesson that many artists have learned and that many are learning today. Finally, it is a lesson that artists are now trying to teach each other, as well as the members of the communities of which they are a part.

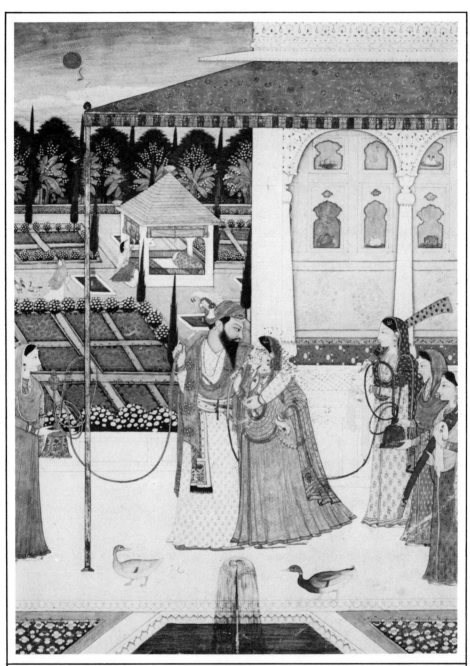

An 18th-century Persian manuscript illustration depicts a woman smoking hashish. According to Persian literature, cannabis was discovered in 1155 by a religious leader who noticed the plant because it did not stand still in the midday heat but danced in the sunlight.

CHAPTER 1

DRUGS: THE LENGTHENING SHADOW

The power of the imagination is the life force of artists. It is no wonder, then, that artists have sought out, experimented with, and cherished those experiences that could fire up, or just expand, that force—a force as old as history.

The earliest artists were influenced and inspired by the forces of nature and the mysteries of their environment. Some of those early influences were the effects on humans of the products of certain plants, among them the hemp plant, cannabis (the hemp plant is classified under the genus *Cannabis*). The hemp plant contained not only fibers to make rope and clothes, but also leaves, seeds, stems, branches, and flowering tops that contained the chemical THC, a substance that is psychoactive. That is, it alters mood, perception, thought processes, and consciousness.

The Lord of Bhang

The hemp plant drug — commonly known as cannabis or marijuana — quickly made its mark in the consciousness of artists. Around 1500 B.C.E. ("before the common era," equivalent to B.C.), the Aryan people invaded India, bringing with them their sacred literature, a collection of four holy books called the *Vedas*. Among the stories in this collection was the tale of the god Siva. According to Indian folklore, Siva brought the marijuana plant down from the Himalayan mountains for the pleasure of the Aryans. He had discovered the cannabis plant while wandering through the fields, sulking after a family fight. Seeking refuge from the burning rays of the sun, Siva ducked under the leaves of cannabis plants. Curious about them, he chewed some of their leaves. The experience so refreshed him that it became his favorite food. The Indians' name for cannabis was bhang, so Siva became known as the Lord of Bhang.

Bhang is also the name of a liquid concoction made from marijuana leaves and a variety of spices, sugar, and milk. The drink became as common in India as alcohol has in the United States. Even in modern times it is often enjoyed on festive occasions. Bhang appears in numerous Indian stories and folksongs. As early as the 10th century C.E. ("common era," equivalent to A.D.), bhang was referred to in Indian literature as the "food of the gods."

In a 16th-century Indian farce called *Dhurtasamagama* (*Rogue's Congress*), two beggars ask an unscrupulous judge

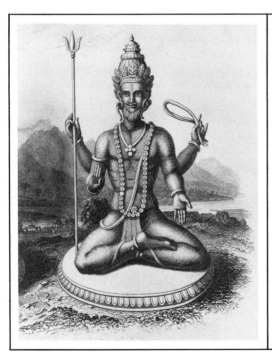

Siva, the god of destruction and reproduction, is one of the main Hindu deities and is credited by Indian folklore as the discoverer of cannabis.

to render a decision on a quarrel they are having. When the judge demands prepayment for his service, one of the beggars offers him some bhang.

The Dancing Plant

The Arabs, too, have a legend that tells how the mind-altering powers of cannabis were discovered. According to their literature, Haydar, the Persian founder of the religious order called Sufis, discovered the plant in 1155 while venturing into the fields after a long, self-imposed confinement in a monastery. He returned from his walk with a strange air of happiness about him and explained to his disciples that he had found a most unusual plant. Unlike the other plants in the field, he said, it did not stand still in the oppressive heat of the day. Rather, it danced about in the sunlight. Curious about the dancing plant, Haydar ate some of its leaves and became euphoric. The leader of the Sufis agreed to show his followers where to find this wondrous plant, but only on the condition that they never reveal the secret to anyone but fellow Sufis.

"The One Thousand and One Nights"

Sometime between 1000 and 1700 a collection of Arab stories grew into the masterpiece now called *The One Thousand and One Nights*. They are stories told by a young harem girl, Scheherazade, to entertain her husband, the sultan Shahriyar. One of these yarns is the "Tale of the Hashish Eater." Hashish is a more potent form of marijuana made from dried and pressed cannabis flowers, leaves, and resin.

The hashish eater squandered his money on hashish and other pleasures. The drug drew him into a dream world in which he was a handsome and wealthy playboy. His hallucinations were characterized by a quality known as "double consciousness," in which the drug taker is aware that he is hallucinating. (This particular state of altered consciousness would come to play a central role in sophisticated 19th-century literature.) The downfall of the hashish eater, as recounted by Scheherazade, came one day when his fellow townspeople, outraged by his chronic intoxication, beat him severely and threw him out of the public bath.

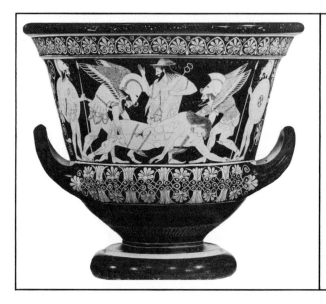

This kylix (drinking cup) from the 6th century B.C.E. depicts the death of Sarpedon, a Greek hero during the Trojan War. Vessels such as this were used in ancient Greece to hold alcoholic drinks.

Against Sorrow

Homer, the great ancient Greek poet who probably lived during the 8th century B.C.E., appears to have been familiar with the soothing effects of some mysterious drug. In his epic work the *Odyssey*, Helen of Troy meets a drug dealer named Polydamna. (In the *Iliad* Homer had told the story of how Helen of Troy had been kidnapped from the Trojans by the Greeks, thus precipitating the Trojan War.) After the war she stops in Egypt with her husband, Menelaus, and there encounters Polydamna, who sells her a drug called *nepenthe* ("against sorrow"). The drug banished sadness, according to Homer, even in the face of the worst personal tragedies. Helen uses the drug years later during a party given by Menelaus. The guests become gloomy when the conversation turns to Menelaus's great friend Odysseus, who has dropped from sight since the war. In order to raise everyone's spirits, Helen slips nepenthe into the guests' wine. Although talk about Odysseus continues, the conversation evokes no further grief from the guests.

Because cannabis was unknown in Egypt until a thousand years after Homer wrote his stories, and opium is mentioned in ancient Egyptian writings, the mysterious nepenthe most likely was opium.

Knowledge of opium's power passed to the Romans as their growing empire enveloped the Greeks. In his epic poem the *Aeneid*, the Roman poet Virgil mentions that opium is a soporific, or a drug that induces drowsiness. The Roman physician Galen used it freely to treat his patients; so revered was this ancient healer that his writings influenced European doctors for many centuries after his death. (Opium grew firmly entrenched in Western medical lore. Its use became commonplace in Europe by the 17th and 18th centuries, and the drug was easily available to the artists of that time.)

The Old Man of the Mountains

During the early Middle Ages, the entire issue of drugs and drug taking was in virtual eclipse. By the end of the 13th century, however, traders from the East were bringing back stories of the effect of drugs on humans, and European interest in psychoactive substances was sparked anew. One such story, told by a trader from Venice held captive in a jail in Genoa during a war between those two Italian cities, showed the dark side of drug use.

The jailed storyteller, who had been seized during a sea battle on his return from the Far East, was Marco Polo. He dictated his stories to a scribe, who preserved his incredible adventures for future readers.

Marco Polo spoke of a ruthless Persian strongman called Hasan-ibn-Sabah, who convinced his followers that he was a divine leader of the Ismaili sect of the Shiite Moslem religion. Hasan lived in his mountain stronghold of Alamut, called the Eagle's Nest. This Old Man of the Mountains, as he was called, kept his bloody group of bandits loyal to him through a devious ploy. A candidate who wished to join his group of terrorists had to take a drug — probably opium — that rendered him unconscious. (Although legend has it that the drug was hashish, one expert points out that there is probably no basis for this belief. Still, some people feel that the word "assassin" is derived from the Arabic word meaning hashish or hashish eaters.) While asleep, the man was carried into a beautiful garden filled with flowers, milk, honey, and beautiful women. When he awoke, he was allowed to partake of all the pleasures of the garden. After enjoying the fruits of paradise he was drugged once again and brought before the Old

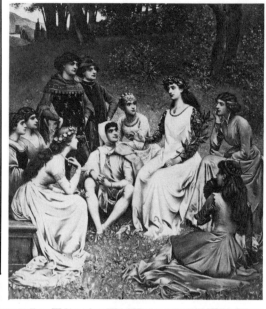

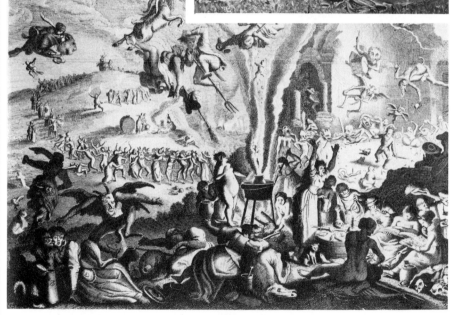

Man. When the candidate awoke and begged to be readmitted to the garden, the Old Man made him first promise that, as a loyal member of the band, he would follow Hasan's orders without question. The Old Man thus was able to recruit a band of fanatical followers eager to rob and murder at his command.

The story of the Old Man of the Mountains was based on a historical figure called Hasan, a Persian chieftain who controlled his men by convincing them that only by following his religious guidance could they achieve paradise.

Tales from the East

There is no evidence that Hasan ever really used drugs to control his men. But the story was picked up by the Italian author Giovanni Boccaccio. In his 14th-century masterpiece, the *Decameron*, Boccaccio refers to a mysterious and marvelous drug that was used by the Old Man of the Mountains when he wanted to send someone to paradise.

By this time, painters were also incorporating drugs into their work. A Persian manuscript from the 14th century, for example, is adorned with a painting of an aristocratic woman smoking hashish with a water pipe. Medieval paintings of the Witches' Sabbath (which were meetings of witches and their worshipers) depicted groups of women stirring some mysterious drug in a large cauldron. In the 15th century, demonologists (people who believed in and studied demons) claimed that one of the most important ingredients of this witches' brew was hemp. In a papal fiat issued in 1484, Pope Innocent VIII condemned both witchcraft and the use of hemp.

There were very few references to cannabis in French literature, travel books, or botanical sources before 1800. That began to change, however, when Napoleon's army occupied Egypt and discovered hashish in the late 18th century. French scientists in Egypt with the invading army began studying and using the drug and sent home samples to their colleagues for further investigation. This action sparked an increased awareness of hallucinatory drugs in Europe.

By 1800, writers, travelers, and scientists, were bringing a steady stream of news of the East to France and England, and such works as *The One Thousand and One Nights* became better known to the reading public. Among those readers most enthralled by these exotic stories was a group of writers, poets, and artists in these two countries who fancied that drugs might be a good way to enhance their creativity.

Drugs had truly arrived in the arts by then. What lay ahead was a long period of use, misuse, and tragedy that continues to this day.

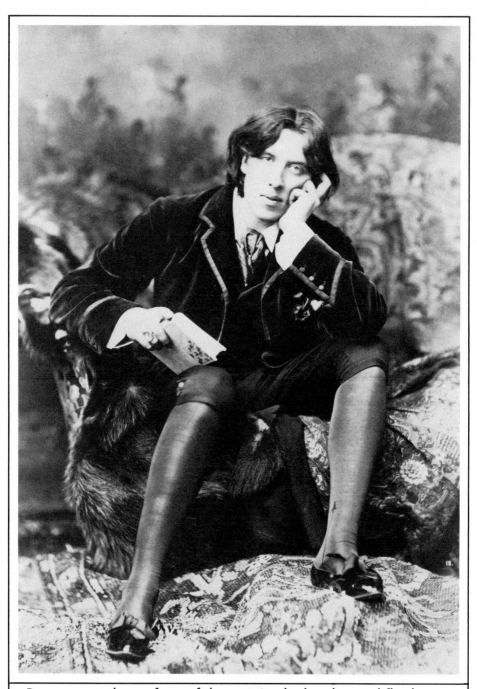

Drugs were only one facet of the notoriously decadent and flamboyant lifestyle of the British writer Oscar Wilde. Both tremendous wit and profound sadness are found in his works.

CHAPTER 2

ROMANTICISM AND DECADENCE

The early and mid-19th century in Europe was a time of experimentation in the arts. During this time, which was known as the Romantic period, the workings of the mind became of great interest, both philosophically and as a potential wellspring of creativity.

Many artists believed that one of the most important creative roles of the brain was its power to synthesize dreams. Those ghostly, fleeting glimpses of another world intrigued writers both in America and abroad and sparked lively conversations among them. Two of the most famous such writers were Samuel Taylor Coleridge and Edgar Allan Poe.

By this time, not only stories of hashish and opium but the drugs themselves were routinely available to artists looking to enrich their dreams with fantastic visions or to experience waking reveries they could incorporate into their works. Opium was particularly easy to come by. It had become a popular "wonder drug" throughout Europe and was readily available at the chemist's shop — the forerunner of the modern pharmacy—for all manner of ills, real or imaginary.

But the free use of opium took a terrible toll, and thousands of people became addicted.

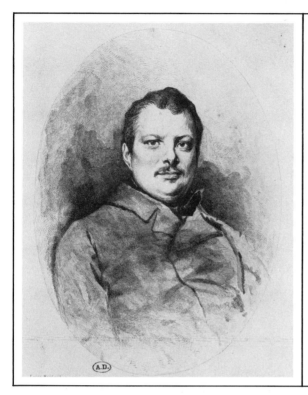

One of the most prolific French authors of all time, Honoré de Balzac was a highly disciplined writer who vehemently condemned drugs for destroying the motivation and will of the artists who used them.

The Hashish Club

During this time, in the mid-19th century, Dr. Jacques-Joseph Moreau, a French psychiatrist, was studying the properties of mental illness by using hashish to inspire hallucinations and induce a "model psychosis" in himself. He extended his studies to a group of painters, poets, and writers who belonged to a club founded by Théophile Gautier. Among its members were the writers Alexandre Dumas (*The Count of Monte Cristo* and *The Three Musketeers*) and Victor Hugo (*Les Misérables* and *The Hunchback of Notre Dame*) and the great Romantic artist Eugène Delacroix. Many members of the Hashish Club, as the group was called, used hashish or opium and wove drug-induced reveries and dreams into their works.

Gautier already knew that such stories would sell. The exotic hashish stories drifting out of the Eastern countries, such as those in *The One Thousand and One Nights*, fascinated European audiences. Gautier's own popular article, "Le Hashish," published in 1843, detailed his hallucinations under the influence of the drug. Gautier later wrote a story based on the Hashish Club.

"Le Club des Hachichins," published in 1846, described the club and its members. Gautier painted a spooky picture of his journey through the fog to the hotel where the club met. Once inside, a mysterious physician offered him some green hashish paste. Gautier then discussed the ancient legend of the Old Man of the Mountains and how the wicked leader of the assassins controlled his fanatical band of killers by giving them hashish.

In "La Pipe d'opium," Gautier described how, during his own opium reveries, he stared at the ceiling as it turned deeper and deeper blue, finally becoming transparent, as it disclosed the star-filled night above.

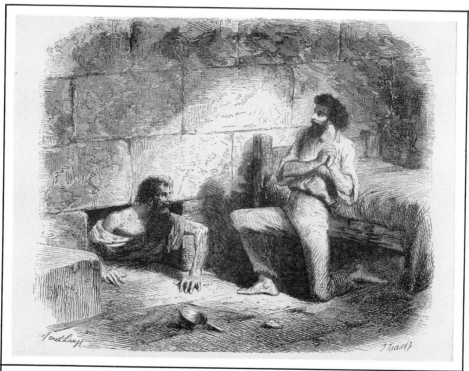

A scene from Alexandre Dumas's classic The Count of Monte Cristo, *which recycled the Old Man of the Mountains tale.*

Eventually, however, Gautier stopped taking drugs. He wrote that a real writer "needs no other than his own natural dreams, and does not care to have his thoughts controlled by the influence of any agency whatever."

Although there is no evidence that Alexandre Dumas used hashish and other drugs heavily, he too recycled the Old Man of the Mountains story. In Dumas's great novel *The Count of Monte Cristo*, the character Franz meets the leader of a band of smugglers, whose headquarters are hidden underground. Franz is led blindfolded down into a sunken palace that is furnished with wondrous articles from around the world — much as candidates for membership in Hasan's tribe were drugged before being carried into a mountain paradise. In the palace, Franz enjoys a sumptuous feast with Sinbad, the bandit leader, who offers him green hashish paste and tells him the story of Hasan.

Synesthesia

Another member of the Hashish Club, Charles Baudelaire, used both opium and hashish. He was a famous and notorious poet, author of the controversial anthology *Les Fleurs du Mal* (*The Flowers of Evil*), first published in 1857. According to Alethea Hayter, author of the book *Opium and the Romantic Imagination*, Baudelaire probably began experimenting with opium while he was a university student at the Sorbonne in France about 1840. Baudelaire and his friends also used marijuana, and an account of the effects of both drugs appears in his book *Paradis artificiels* (*Artificial Paradises*).

In the first part of this book, Baudelaire describes in detail his own experiences and discussions with his fellow writers on the mental effects of hashish. The writers compared how hashish influenced their reactions to music, lights, colors, clock faces, frescoes on the walls and ceilings of rooms, and other objects and experiences.

One of the effects of hashish that the Romantic writers cherished most was the phenomenon called *synesthesia* — a correspondence between one sense and another. Alethea Hayter writes in her book, for example, that Edgar Allan Poe claimed that he was simultaneously aware of both the buzzing of a gnat and the orange ray of the light spectrum. Gautier experienced musical notes from a piano as sparks of red and blue. Baudelaire himself experienced the mental transformation of musical notes into arithmetical calculations.

Hayter suggests that some of the synesthetic experiences of the Romantic writers were caused by hashish or opium, but that some were probably also due to the natural powers of the imagination of the poetic mind.

Despite his experiments with drugs, Baudelaire was wary of both hashish and opium and believed that "it is the nature of hashish to weaken the will . . . to bestow imagination without the power to make use of it." In a more pointed warning, he wrote, "Think of the frightful state of a man whose paralyzed imagination can no longer work without the help of hashish or opium."

Baudelaire graphically portrayed the horrors of opium in his prose poem "La Chambre double," which seems to be based on personal experience. Baudelaire wrote of lying on a bed in a filthy room with dirty, dilapidated furniture, a cold, cheerless fireplace plastered with spittle, grimy, rain-streaked windows, and air gone stale with smoke and other stenches. His flask of laudanum, a mixture of opium and wine, is the sole object of comfort to him.

The prolific French novelist Honoré de Balzac, who chronicled the society of his time in his multivolume novel *The Human Comedy*, was even more emphatic about drug use by artists, although he did sample hashish at a meeting of the Hashish Club. Gautier wrote that Balzac believed there is no greater shame or suffering than for people to renounce control over their own will.

The Torment of Addiction

As in France, people in Britain used opium both medically and recreationally in the beginning of the 19th century. But the publication in 1821 of Thomas De Quincey's book *Confessions of an English Opium Eater* created a sensation. Here for the first time was a detailed description of a writer's involvement with opium and the torment of addiction that cast a pall over much of the author's personal and creative life.

A highly revised French translation of *Confessions* inspired the composer Hector Berlioz to create *Symphonie fantastique*, a musical fantasy about a young musician haunted by a woman's face wherever he goes. In despair of ever gaining her love, he attempts to poison himself with opium. The musician survives but has a horrible vision that he has murdered his beloved, and is being carried in a solemn procession to his execution.

De Quincey's description of the effects of opium, so graphically described in *Confessions*, appears as a summarized translation into French as the second part of Baudelaire's *Paradis artificiels*. Baudelaire merely added a comment or two on De Quincey's character and style: according to Hayter, Baudelaire believed that De Quincey's *Confessions* was the most definitive statement on the subject of opium addiction.

The original *Confessions* is an elegant example of how artists integrated into their work both their personal reality and their drug-induced dreams and reveries. De Quincey's

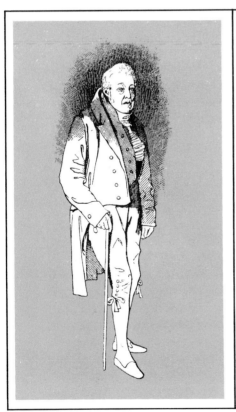

Samuel Taylor Coleridge, the revered Romantic poet who composed the epic poem Kubla Khan, *was hobbled during his later years by a tragic opium addiction.*

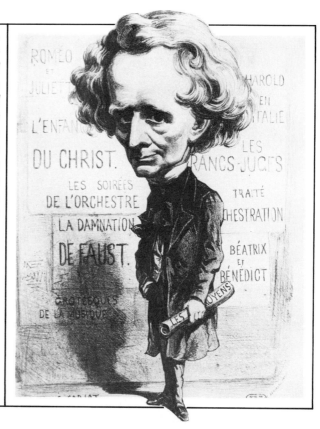

A caricature of the composer Hector Berlioz, whose musical fantasy Symphonie fantastique *was based loosely upon a highly revised French translation of Thomas De Quincey's famous diary of drug addiction,* Confessions of an English Opium Eater.

reality was grim indeed. Starting in his youth in the late 1700s and continuing into adulthood, he suffered an extraordinary series of personal losses due to illness, including his sister Elizabeth, who had been a close companion, his father, and later, two of his sons, his uncle, his wife, and his friend Samuel Taylor Coleridge. It was while De Quincey was at Oxford University that he began to take opium, at first to relieve digestive pain, but then to experience the drug's pleasures. By 1813 he was addicted.

According to *Confessions*, De Quincey had dreams that were accompanied by "deep-seated anxiety and melancholy, such as are wholly incommunicable by words." He wrote of descending each night into "chasms and sunless abysses, depths below depths," from which he did not escape by waking up. Opium was entwined in his nightmares, thoughts, fears, obsessions (including his obsession with the legend of the Old Man of the Mountains), and much of his writing.

Vision of Sudden Death

A typical example of this integration of reality and unreality under the force of opium appears in De Quincey's *The English Mail Coach*, a three-part prose poem about a journey in a mail coach through the English countryside. In part, it celebrates the author's hope of escaping from opium addiction. But the third part, "The Vision of Sudden Death," is based on De Quincey's actual experience one night in a mail coach during a trip from his home in Manchester in 1816 or 1817.

De Quincey, who was under the influence of opium, realized the driver had fallen asleep. As the horses clattered on out of control, De Quincey saw a small cart carrying a young couple coming the other way. The driver of the cart barely managed to pull over to the side of the road before the coach swept by. De Quincey, who had been unable to react quickly enough to blow a warning on the carriage horn, watched as the young man's terrified lover threw her hands into the air and screamed in terror.

When De Quincey wrote about that scene in "The Vision of Sudden Death," the runaway vehicle became a ghostly coach rushing at midnight into a vast cathedral, pounding along its floor toward a city of tombstones rising up in the distance. As the carriage hurtles through the aisle of the vast cathedral, it bears down on a small cart carrying a young girl. Just before the coach careens into the cart, a stone trumpeter, carved into a tomb, comes to life and, with a blast of his horn, warns the girl of the impending collision. The blast carries the girl to an altar high up in the cathedral amid a beam of crimson light, as the first rays of dawn pierce the gloom of the night.

Despite such imaginative writing, De Quincey had no illusions about opium's ability to enrich the imagination. In fact, he wrote in *Confessions* that opium produced interesting dreams only if the dreamer had an interesting mind. If a man who talks only of oxen takes opium, he wrote, that man will dream only of oxen.

Like his friend Thomas De Quincey, Samuel Taylor Coleridge was tormented by nightmares, which became more horrible after he began to abuse opium. Like De Quincey, Coleridge derived some of his material from opium reveries. He wrote that he spent three hours in a chair in a "sleep of external senses," composing 200 to 300 lines of what became

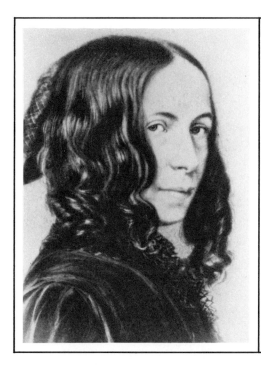

Elizabeth Barrett Browning was both the wife of the Romantic poet Robert Browning and a noted poet in her own right. She used morphine for medical purposes but never succumbed to addiction.

the poem *Kubla Khan*. But as Hayter points out in her book, it was his enormous intellect, education, and memory that permitted Coleridge to construct that poem from the words and visions of his reverie. And Coleridge wrote *Kubla Khan* during his early experiments with opium, before addiction began to hobble his mind.

Along with De Quincey, Coleridge seems to have seen to the heart of opium's destructive potential. Coleridge composed his poem "Dejection" as a recognition of mental faculties lost forever, dulled into oblivion by opium. His poem "The Pains of Sleep" represents the horrors experienced during advanced opium addiction. And in the fragment of an unfinished poem, he refers to the trap of opium as a limbo that is

> wall'd round, and made a spirit-jail secure,
> By the mere horror of blank Naught-at-all.

Of course, other artists took opium for various reasons but escaped addiction. Elizabeth Barrett Browning, for example, took morphine, a derivative of opium, from 1837 to 1845 to relieve the pain of a spinal ailment that plagued her

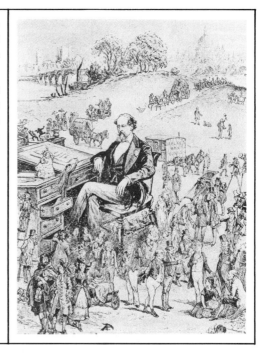

An illustration of Charles Dickens depicts the most famous of all Victorian novelists surrounded by a gallery of his characters. Dickens expressed through his novels the customs and injustices of Victorian society, and he included London's opium dens in his descriptions.

all her life. A reviewer at the time commented that a reader could well wonder whether her poem " A Rhapsody of Life's Progress," in which she described various bizarre images, was written under the influence of opium. Browning did not succumb to the temptations of opium abuse, however, and never became an addict.

Though he did not become addicted, Charles Dickens also used opium for medical reasons. In his last novel, *The Mystery of Edwin Drood*, Dickens created the character of John Jaspers, an addict who frequents London opium dens. Dickens himself actually toured these dens to get background material for the novel. He described in this story an old woman whom he had seen using an opium pipe that had been made out of an ink bottle.

The American Scene

The publication in England of *Confessions* had made opium a common prop in American as well as European literature.

Opium figured prominently in many works of Edgar Allan Poe, who was a heavy drinker and opium user. The main characters in "Tale of the Ragged Mountains" and "Ligeia" are addicts. In one of Poe's masterpieces, "The Fall of the House of Usher," a traveler seeing Roderick Usher's bleak house for the first time compares the experience to coming out of an opium trance and back to reality "with an utter depression of soul. . . . There was an iciness, a sinking, a sickening of the heart—an unredeemed dreariness of thought."

In the story Usher himself suffered from an affliction called *hyperaesthesia*, a "morbid acuteness of the senses" that made stong tastes, smells, bright light, and any music except faint stringed instruments unendurable to him. It is probable that Poe, who was himself a heavy opium user, suffered similar symptoms.

In 19th-century America hemp was still considered by most people to be simply a valuable agricultural crop for its raw material, which was used to make rope. References to the psychoactive properties of the plant were relatively few. John Greenleaf Whittier's 1854 antislavery poem, "The Haschish," however, contrasted the enslavement of individuals by hashish with the enslavement of a whole race by the cotton industry.

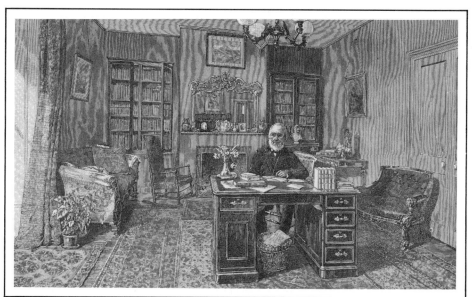

In his work "The Haschish," 19th-century poet John Greenleaf Whittier compared the plight of addiction to the enslavement of an entire race.

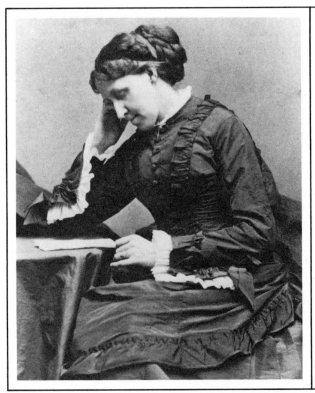

Louisa May Alcott, whose most famous novel, Little Women, *is still widely read, described the effects of marijuana in her short story "Perilous Play."*

In addition, Bayard Taylor's writings about the Middle and Far East introduced many Americans to hashish. Not surprisingly, he wrote about the legend of the Old Man of the Mountains in the introduction of his book *Land of the Saracens*, one of many works that chronicled his worldwide travels.

Another reference to the psychoactive properties of the hemp plant was provided by Louisa May Alcott, who described the effects of marijuana in her short story "Perilous Play." And Thomas Bailey Aldrich wrote in his poem "Hascheesh" of marijuana's initially pleasurable effects, which turned into a monstrous nightmare after he continued to use the drug.

The Decadent Era

By 1840 the Romantic era had begun to wane, supplanted by a vision of art animating a new group of artists in England and France. These artists took literally Théophile Gautier's dictum, "art for art's sake." They rejected morality as an important element in their work and emphasized the supremacy of form over content in art. For this reason, they became known as "decadents," a term derived from *décadents*, originally applied to a group of French post-Romantic poets and prose writers.

Like their Romantic forebears, the decadents sought inspiration and escape from boredom through drugs. William Butler Yeats, the great Irish poet and playwright, used hashish as well as the hallucinatory drug mescaline, which is the psychoactive ingredient of the mescal cactus. Havelock Ellis, the psychologist, physician, poet, and essayist, also used mescaline. Ernest Dowson, whose poetry voiced regret for the passing of youth and beauty, denial of love, and rejection of pleasure, gave up hashish but became an alcoholic.

Oscar Wilde, the witty Irish playwright and leader of the decadent movement in England, preferred absinthe, a toxic

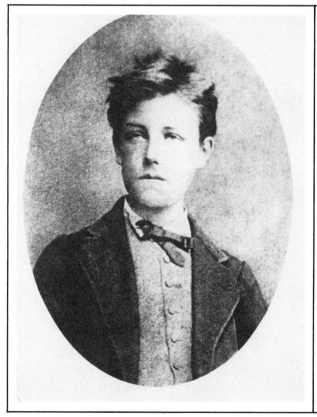

Arthur Rimbaud pushed himself to the physical and emotional limits of suffering with the help of drugs and alcohol. Far from aiding his creativity, his excesses forced him to abandon his art before the age of 20.

liqueur distilled from wormwood, angelica root, and other aromatic woods and steeped in alcohol. A strong drink, it is 70% to 80% alcohol. Most Western countries eventually outlawed its manufacture and sale, but it was very popular during the decadent era.

In France, the post-Romantic poet Arthur Rimbaud became a leading light of that country's decadent milieu. He and his roustabout companion, the poet Paul Verlaine, consumed both absinthe and hashish. The two traveled and lived together at various times and eventually fought violently with each other. Alcohol sparked Rimbaud's creative drive, but it also loosened his sarcastic tongue, with which he alienated many acquaintances.

Rimbaud's life and works reflect his disenchantment with society, religion, and even poetry. He was born Jean-Arthur Rimbaud in 1854 to an adventurer father and a mother who treated him severely. His parents had little use for each other, and usually lived apart. A brilliant child, Rimbaud, who was raised by his religious mother, excelled in school, and at age 12 had a burning faith and piety. As he grew, he widened his horizons from Latin literature to the writings of Baudelaire, among other authors.

Derangement of the Senses

Rimbaud's demanding genius eventually turned him into a rebel. Bored with his life in the French countryside and feeling the need to experience new things, Rimbaud ran away to Paris at the age of 15. Soon afterwards he began his association with Verlaine.

During his time in Paris, Rimbaud began experimenting with drugs. He believed that a poet must make himself a "seer" not only through self-debauchery and suffering, but also through derangement of the senses: "He exhausts all the poisons within himself and retains only their quintessence," Rimbaud wrote.

The poet often returned to his mother's home to rest and compose himself. During one of these visits his mother was startled to hear strange sounds coming from her son, who had locked himself in his room. There, alone, he scribbled out, amid sobs, cries of anger, and curses, one of his classic works, *Une Saison en enfer* (*A Season in Hell*).

This autobiographical prose poem describes the tortured spiritual conflict raging within Rimbaud: the battles between damnation and salvation, between heroism and greed, between self-denial and the intoxicating lure of evil. The battle begins early in the piece.

> One evening I set Beauty on my knees—And I
> found her sour—
> And I cursed her.
> I took arms against justice. . . .
> I was able to obliterate from my mind all human
> hope. Upon each joy, to strangle it, I made
> the soundless spring of a wild beast.

For Rimbaud, this work would be his last. In order to become a seer he had abused himself with alcohol, hashish, and cynical degeneracy. Finally, he rejected his art. He left the world of poetry and disappeared into the world of city streets, railroad stations, and seaports. He was 19 years old.

Rimbaud left behind him a copy of his last work. A Belgian company had put it into print, but the poet lost interest in it and refused to pay for the printing. *A Season in Hell* simply collected dust until a Belgian book lover came upon it in the print shop in 1901.

Leaving Europe behind, Rimbaud toured the Mediterranean and Mideast, including the area of the Red Sea. Eventually he settled in Africa, where he worked as a businessman for much of the remainder of his life. Rimbaud died in 1891 at the age of 37.

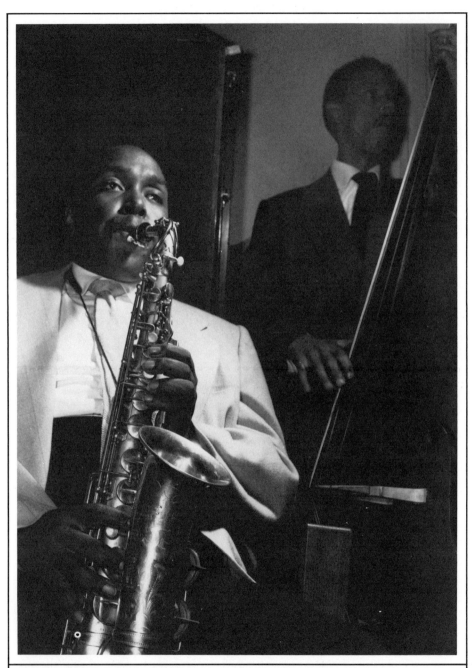

Charlie "Bird" Parker (left), one of the greatest saxophone players of all time, originated the rhythmic and harmonic variation of jazz called "bop." Tragically, Parker was addicted to both heroin and alcohol and died in 1955 at the age of 35.

CHAPTER 3

DRUGS AND JAZZ

In the early 20th century, about a million Americans, many of them upright citizens from small towns, were living lives of quiet addiction to opium and morphine. A home remedy for many years, opium use was widely accepted, and addiction was not generally looked upon as degenerate or criminal. Alcohol, too, was a very popular drug in turn-of-the-century America. Cannabis was still relatively unknown at this time, used only by a few writers and artists, and for some medicinal purposes.

In 1914, Congress passed the Harrison Act, a measure that forced narcotics users to obtain their drugs through pharmacists, who, in turn, had to pay for a tax stamp. Because other people could not buy these stamps, opium, its derivatives, and cocaine were effectively outlawed unless prescribed by a physician. Five years later, Congress enacted the 18th Amendment, which outlawed the consumption and sale of all alcohol. Prohibition was a national law until it was repealed in 1933.

The Harrison Act and Prohibition were manifestations of a reformist spirit abroad in the America of that time that took exception not only to the "vices" of drug and alcohol abuse, but also to such "low" pastimes as smoking and dancing. The reformers took aim at such "lewd" dances as the tango, hesitation waltz, turkey trot, and Charleston. A new form of music also scandalized these guardians of public morals. Its rhythms suggested loose morals and low life. It was born in the harmonies of black spirituals, work songs, and hymns and grew up in New Orleans brothels, where it entertained the ladies and their gentleman patrons. The music was different. It was American. It was racy. It was jazz.

Musicians and Marijuana

The black musicians of the New Orleans brothels smoked marijuana to help them play jazz through the long hours; some thought their music sounded better under the influence of "moota," as the drug was called in this part of the city.

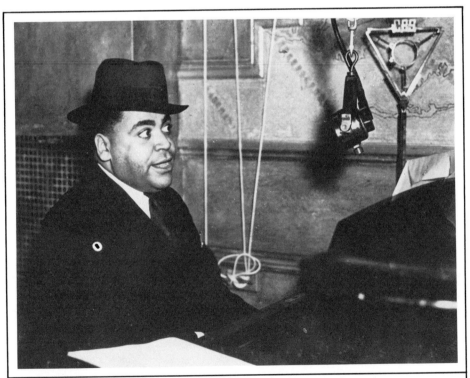

Fats Waller makes a radio broadcast. Waller, a jazz pianist, wrote many hit songs in the 1940s. But the strains of touring, aggravated by alcohol abuse, precipitated his premature death.

In the 1930s a white jazz clarinetist named Milton Mezzrow moved from Chicago to New York and began packaging and selling thick marijuana cigarettes, which became so popular that "mezz" became a synonym for marijuana, and a well-packed marijuana cigarette was called a "mezzrole."

As jazz spread its rhythms across the nation, the image of the marijuana-smoking jazz musician and listener became part of the cultural scene. In the 1930s "reefer" songs, pieces referring to marijuana cigarettes, became popular among jazz musicians. Generally these songs were written by black musicians for black audiences and were unknown to most people ouside the jazz world. Some of these early marijuana songs include Cab Calloway's "That Funny Reefer Man" and Fats Waller's "Viper's Moan" ("viper" was the word for a person who used marijuana). Even the popular white musician Benny Goodman contributed a song, "Sweet Marijuana Brown."

By now, drugs of all types were not only part of the jazz scene — they were changing it. As drugs victimized jazz artists, the jazz world lost the musical contributions these artists could have made. One of those lost artists was Charlie "Bird" Parker, the great saxophonist and composer of "bop," a form of jazz with a more elaborate rhythm structure than classical jazz and an emphasis on harmony rather than melody. Parker died in 1955 at the age of 35 after many years of addiction to heroin and alcohol. Some jazz artists were luckier. They survived, although their lives were wracked and wasted by drugs.

By the mid-1930s, jazz had already bopped across the Atlantic and was entertaining enthusiastic audiences in Europe. Unfortunately, as jazz became more widespread in Europe, so did marijuana. In February 1936 the English music magazine *Melody Maker* carried an exposé on marijuana use by British musicians, reporting with alarm that use of the drug was spreading rapidly among them.

The Dark Underworld

Unfortunately, newspaper articles about marijuana abuse did not curb the increasing use of drugs among jazz musicians. In 1941 a 15-year-old jazz saxophonist named Art Pepper was already a heavy drinker. Music was his escape from the traumas of a broken home, and drugs gave him relief from his craving for affection, his anger, and his self-doubt.

Pepper married at 17 and, while on tour with a jazz band, started taking heroin. He spent much of the next 16 years in prison for narcotics convictions, and eventually his wife divorced him. He remarried, but his second wife, after becoming suicidal over his drug use, became an addict as well. The marriage fell apart. Pepper managed to keep working for a while, and even recorded some albums. But the draw of dope was too strong. He could not find enough work to support his habit, so he sold his instruments and other possessions. With nothing left to sell, he turned to burglary and remained for years in the dark underworld of addiction. Eventually he checked into a drug rehabilitation center. In 1977 he made his first public reappearance at the Newport Jazz Festival in Newport, Rhode Island. He went on tour after that appearance, although he still suffered from liver damage caused by years of alcohol abuse.

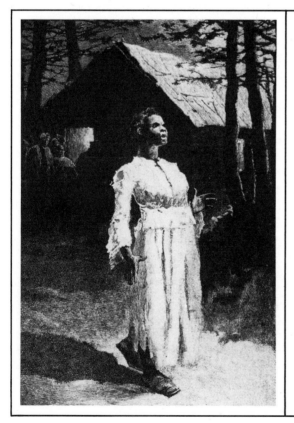

A 19th-century engraving depicts a spiritual singer at a Negro settlement. Spirituals, which were first developed by American slaves, were one of several influences on early jazz styles.

A Frightening Thing to Watch

It should be noted that in 1957 the problem of drug use among jazz musicians prompted serious discussion among members of a special panel at the Newport Jazz Festival. The panel was composed of a jazz drummer, a piano player, a lawyer, a psychologist, a priest, and two jazz critics. Their discussion of the topic "Music and the Use of Habituating and Addicting Drugs" was historic. The world of jazz was facing one of the biggest threats to the welfare of its musicians.

One of the panel members, John Hammond, the preeminent record producer, emphasized that musicians had to bear some of the blame for the stigma of narcotics on the world of jazz. He pointed out that jazz musicians had taken drugs for years, and some, like Milton Mezzrow, had become dealers. Many jazz musicians had written songs about drugs and glamorized their use, leading the young, up-and-coming musicians to think that it was "cool" to use these chemicals.

One of the most damaging myths about drugs and jazz, according to Hammond, was that they help spark the musician's creative drive. It might stimulate, Hammond warned, but it hurts the timing. Drugs wreaked havoc not only on the player's technical ability, he pointed out, but also on his personality.

"It's a terrible thing to see talent stifled by narcotics," said panel member Billy Taylor, the great jazz pianist. "It's a frightening thing to watch."

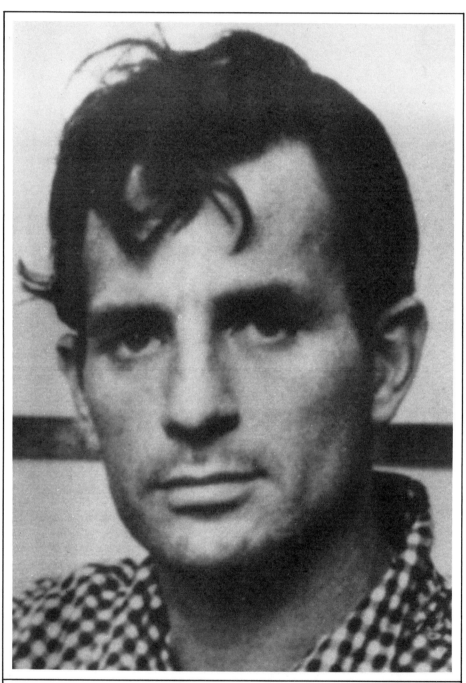

Jack Kerouac, whose novel about underground culture, On The Road, *became the testament of the Beat movement, experimented heavily with psychoactive drugs and died of their long-term effects in 1969.*

CHAPTER 4

DRUGS AND MODERN LITERATURE

The inventive form of music known as jazz lent its name to an entire era; the "jazz age" was a time not only of new trends in dance and music, but also of a certain experimentation in fiction. Writers identified with this period, F. Scott Fitzgerald among them, styled themselves spokesmen for a "lost generation," adrift in a world where traditional standards of morality and behavior no longer applied.

Himself an alcoholic, Fitzgerald created a world of rootless, debauched, morally bankrupt men and women. His first novel, *This Side of Paradise*, is an extended study in disintegration. It is the story of Amory Blaine, a sensitive young man who, after an idyllic childhood, cannot cope with the demands of the adult world. *The Great Gatsby* describes the rise and fall of a bootlegger who attempts to overcome his solitude through a series of lavish parties and is finally destroyed by his one unfulfilled desire, an unrequited passion for a woman. *Tender Is the Night* is the cynical history of the breakdown of a young doctor, destroyed by his impossible obsession with his unstable wife.

The characters in these three novels and in his other works reflect the conflicts and turmoil within Fitzgerald, a gifted but disillusioned author whose life was marked by early success, a debilitating marriage, and, perhaps most tragically, rapid artistic decline caused by a fatal addiction to alcohol.

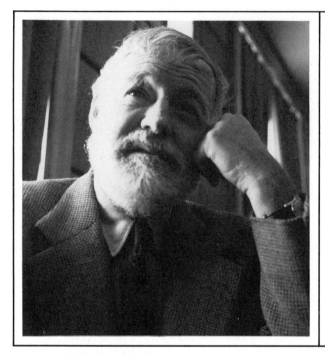

Ernest Hemingway, one of the principal writers of the "lost generation," celebrated the heroism of the individual confronting a hostile world. A heavy drinker, Hemingway frequently associated the use of alcohol with virility in the portrayal of his heroes.

The Surrealists

Many artists, such as Fitzgerald and Ernest Hemingway — another hard-drinking novelist — moved overseas in the 1920s, leaving the moralism of America behind. Ahead lay the Depression and World War II, which put an end to the carefree jazz age and the world as Fitzgerald knew it. These expatriate artists encountered and were influenced by French painters and writers who were in turn immersed in the creative ferment of the surrealist movement, which began around 1924. (The painters associated with this movement will be discussed in Chapter 7.)

Surrealism depended on "free association," or on images derived from the subconscious through spontaneous thought. Its forebears were French poets such as Baudelaire and Rimbaud, and the Italian painter Giorgio de Chirico. This artist greatly influenced surrealism by painting works with faceless figures and exaggerated proportions, creating an unreal, dreamlike quality.

One of the leading surrealists was Jean Cocteau, the great French writer, visual artist, and film maker. Born outside Paris in 1889, Cocteau admired the precocious artistic powers of Baudelaire and Rimbaud. When he was about 30, he met and befriended the novelist and poet Raymond Radiguet, who was then 19. Radiguet was a heavy drinker, and his excesses weakened him, making him particularly vulnerable to disease. When the young writer died of typhus just short of his 21st birthday, Cocteau sank into a deep depression that he treated with opium. He became addicted and spent 60 days in a sanitarium. Cocteau was to smoke opium for the rest of his life, occasionally entering a sanitarium to seek a "cure" (temporary rehabilitation) from his dependence.

Cocteau later wrote that getting up in the morning during the first few months of his addiction was "like being thrown back into dirty water and made to swim." He described his "flight into opium" as a "flight into sickness."

During a "cure" that took place in 1928, Cocteau kept a journal of his experiences. It was later published (in 1930) under the title *Opium: A Diary of Cure*, and was reminiscent

The French surrealist author Jean Cocteau battled opium addiction for much of his life. Alienation and nightmare visions are hallmarks of his artistic vision.

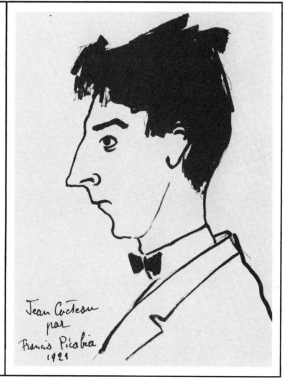

of Thomas De Quincey's autobiographical work, *Confessions of an English Opium Eater.* Toward the end of his treatment, he also began work on his celebrated novel, *Les Enfants terribles (The Bad Children),* the story of a young brother and sister alienated from the adult world and destined to meet a tragic fate.

The Beat Movement

The posture of alienation adopted by writers like Cocteau would have a profound influence on a later generation of artists in America. As the United States entered the 1950s, the country was prospering. Unemployment was at an all-time low, the economy was booming, and the general spirit of the times was one of optimism and an unbridled faith in progress and possibility.

In any free society, however, there are critics and dissenters, and this was certainly the case in the United States of the late 1940s and 1950s. During this time a growing

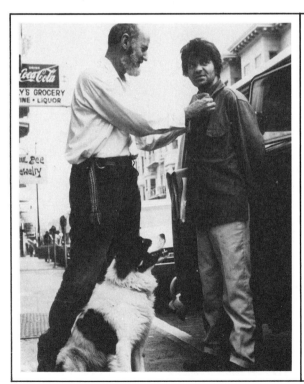

Beat poets Lawrence Ferlinghetti (left) and Gregory Corso converse on a San Francisco street corner. Ferlinghetti's publishing company, City Lights, printed many of the classics of the Beat movement.

coterie of young writers, who gathered in the smoky, cramped jazz clubs and coffeehouses of postwar New York and other large cities, searched for new ways to express their feelings and experiences. Drawing heavily on the legacy of the surrealists and the decadents as well as on the then fashionable pronouncements of the French existentialists, the Beats sought to express their dissatisfaction with what they saw as a complacent, narrow-minded society obsessed with conformity and the success ethic.

The members of the Beat movement were highly vocal in the 1950s, and their influence was felt well into the 1960s. Their romantic militancy against many of the values of American society found expression in the works of authors whose prose reflected their hectic, spontaneous, intense lifestyles. Eastern religions, drugs, new sexual experiences, new places, new faces, and the rejection of convention all fed into the movement's creative cauldron. The true Beat artists provided the intellectual and aesthetic underpinnings of the cult known as the beatniks, a term coined around the time of the Soviet Union's successful launch of the Sputnik satellite in 1957.

The "Disease of Overlife"

Among the leading figures of the Beat movement were the novelists Jack Kerouac and William Burroughs and the poets Allen Ginsberg and Lawrence Ferlinghetti, whose City Lights publishing house in San Francisco brought out many of the major works of the literary movement of which he was a leader.

Kerouac was born in 1922 in Pawtucketville, a French-Canadian community in Lowell, Massachusetts, and spoke French as his first language. Although he entered Columbia University, he never graduated. His early years out of Columbia were characterized by an unfocused but lusty involvement in the series of experiences that life threw his way. He worked for a while as a sportswriter on a newspaper, traveled in the merchant marines, was tossed in a New York jail for being a material witness to a murder, was married and divorced within two months, and began his career as a writer. Early in his writing career Kerouac used amphetamines to help him write but complained to Ginsberg that the drugs made him intellectually "flabby."

In 1950 Kerouac published his first novel, *The Town and the City*. The book described his turbulent relationship with his father, who had died of cancer in 1946, and the sorrow and rootlessness that Kerouac experienced afterward.

Despite the publication of his first book, Kerouac's restless nature left him feeling very much at loose ends in New York. Taking up with a kindred spirit and fellow self-styled vagabond named Neal Cassady, the two set off for Mexico City to meet William Burroughs. There, Kerouac began to smoke marijuana and use morphine, heroin, and peyote. The shadow of Arthur Rimbaud, the manic French decadent writer, fell across Kerouac's life during these hectic early years of his career. The frenetic American author even wrote of Rimbaud as being consumed "by the disease of overlife."

But Kerouac began to fall into the trap of drug addiction himself. In 1952, depressed over the early public failure of his writing, he began to inject heroin several times a week while living in Mexico with Burroughs. Needless to say, the drug only deepened his despair over his lack of success as a writer. But he was determined to start work on a new novel about his childhood in Lowell. Because Burroughs's home was so cramped, Kerouac worked on the book, *Doctor Sax*, in a bathroom.

His mind ravaged by heroin and marijuana, Kerouac, like Rimbaud, experienced derangement of the senses as he pounded out his story — isolated, impoverished, and anonymous.

If Jack Kerouac's career had ended with *Doctor Sax*, he might indeed have remained an irrelevant literary figure. But in 1957 he published a novel that he had completed six years earlier. The book, *On the Road*, became the testament of the Beat movement. The raw spontaneity of its prose reflected a belief in the artistic truth of unrefined human emotion. *On the Road* depicted the underground culture that had rejected the middle-class values of the 1950s and described the sense of release and joy that the less constricted members of society experienced through free-spirited living, travel, sex, drugs, and the expression of intense emotions.

However seriously *On the Road* was or was not taken as literature, it undoubtedly won for itself a lasting place as a cultural artifact. Kerouac lived long enough to become a hero to many young readers who were growing up in the

1960s. But the "disease of overlife" that he had ascribed to Rimbaud caught up with him in 1969, and he died in Florida of a stomach condition caused by alcoholism, drug abuse, and malnutrition.

Allen Ginsberg was another member of the new generation mythologized in *On the Road*. He was an integral member of the Beat movement and a friend of both Kerouac and Burroughs. Ginsberg, who has won a measure of genuine literary prestige that eluded Kerouac, was portrayed in the latter's novel *The Town and the City* as a Rimbaud-like poet named Levinsky.

Born in 1926 in Newark, New Jersey, Ginsberg is the son of a lyric poet who taught high school and college English classes. Ginsberg's mother was psychologically unstable, and her anxiety and paranoia greatly affected her sensitive son.

Ginsberg entered Columbia University in 1943 but was forced to drop out to seek psychiatric help. Although Ginsberg enjoyed literature, he rejected the poetry of his day. His mind searched for new, freer means of expression. Not surprisingly, perhaps, among the writers whose work he studied was Rimbaud. Once out of Columbia he was forced to find work as a welder, night porter, and dishwasher. He met the ordinary people on the street, learned their language, and understood their ways.

Like Kerouac, he shipped out on a merchant marine vessel. Unlike Kerouac, he eventually returned to Columbia and graduated. But Ginsberg was hopeless and fearful about his future, and this negativity, along with his exposure to the street life of New York City, exacerbated his restless nature and drove him more and more to drug use. He was encouraged in his irrational and impetuous behavior by a group of like-minded friends, Neal Cassady among them.

Eventually he took up with Herbert Huncke, a rootless and poor street criminal who introduced Ginsberg and his friend William Burroughs to morphine and the underworld of New York City. Ginsberg eventually found himself in the middle of a wild car chase, as his underworld friends fled from the police in an automobile filled with stolen merchandise. Ginsberg avoided jail by entering a psychiatric hospital for treatment.

The years of drugs, despair, street life, and desperate searches for his own identity found expression in his poetry.

In the poem "Paterson" he wrote:

> I would rather go mad, gone down the dark road
> to Mexico, heroin dripping in my veins,
> eyes and ears full of marijuana,
> eating the god Peyote on the floor of a mudhut on
> the border. . .

"Lysergic Acid," a poem named after the hallucinogenic drug LSD, calls up visions of a demon.

> It is a multiple million eyed monster
> it is hidden in all its elephants and selves
> it hummeth in the electric typewriter
> it is electricity connected to itself . . .

That poem appears in a 1961 volume called *Kaddish and Other Poems, 1958–1960*, which was, in part, an elegy to the suffering of his mother. (The word Kaddish refers to a Judaic mourner's prayer for the dead.)

In 1955, Ginsberg gave a public reading of his poem "Howl" to a San Francisco audience, whose wild enthusiasm for his performance transformed Ginsberg into a "legend" overnight. At the reading, Ginsberg intoned: "I saw the best minds of my generation destroyed by madness. . . ." He described his generation as starving, hysterical, naked beings, dragging themselves through the streets, "looking for an angry fix," and as "angelheaded hipsters burning for the ancient heavenly connection to the starry dynamo in the machinery of night," a reference to the use of drugs by members of the Beat movement as they floated "across the tops of cities contemplating jazz."

The audience reacted passionately to the power and brilliance of his delivery. "Howl" was a record of the despair and desperation of his generation of artists, but it offered the promise of cultural change. The poem not only established Ginsberg as an important poet, but was also a blow for artistic freedom and the first important public proclamation of the Beat movement.

The Darkest Side of Drugs

Like Kerouac and Ginsberg, William Burroughs used drugs, and there are references to drugs in his works. But unlike his two fellow Beat artists, Burroughs was addicted to heroin

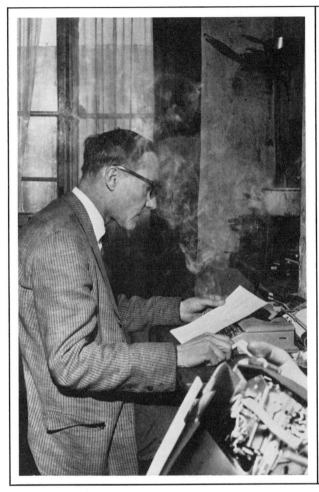

Although the works of William Burroughs describe the full horror of drug addiction and withdrawal, during the 1960s the writer was lionized by young people who themselves glamorized the effects of drugs.

and morphine for many years. Like Rimbaud, he came from a rather aristocratic family. His mother was a direct descendant of Robert E. Lee, the commanding general of the Confederate Army, and his grandfather, William Seward Burroughs, was the famous inventor who founded the office machine and computer company that bore his name before it merged with another company in 1986.

Burroughs graduated from Harvard University and later moved to New York, where he met Kerouac and Ginsberg. (Burroughs eventually went into self-exile, and lived for many years in Mexico, North Africa, and Europe before returning to the United States.) His drug addiction provided the basis for his first novel, *Junkie* (published in 1953), in which he describes the pusher in starkly unromantic terms:

> This man walks around in the places where he once exercised his obsolete and unthinkable trade. But he is unperturbed. His eyes are black with an insect's unseeing calm. . . . What is his lost trade? Definitely of a servant class and something to do with the dead, though he is not an embalmer. . . . He is as specialized as an insect, for the performance of some inconceivably vile function.

With his notorious novel *Naked Lunch*, which he began in 1955 and published in 1959, Burroughs contributed a lasting memorial to the darkest side of drugs and his own drug addiction. The novel traces the hallucinatory horror of his withdrawal from drugs, during which he imagines that New York City is in ruins, and huge centipedes and scorpions crawl in and out of empty bars, cafeterias, and drugstores.

Twelve years after *Naked Lunch* appeared, Burroughs published *The Wild Boys*, a novel about a band of fanatical, hashish-eating young criminals set during the last decades of the 20th century. The theme is borrowed from the legend of the Old Man of the Mountains that Marco Polo brought back from the Far East hundreds of years before, and that writers throughout the centuries have recycled time and again.

The Loss of Allure

When the Beat writers were at the height of their fame and creative intensity, drug use in American society was far from the mainstream scourge it was to become hardly more than a decade later. For the Beats, the romanticization of drugs was as much as anything else an aspect of their self-conscious nonconformity with regard to every aspect of "bourgeois" American society. Glorifying drugs was but one of several ways writers like Kerouac and Burroughs could announce their utter separation from, and contempt for, the America of their time.

However, as drug use became a more and more routine ingredient of ordinary American life itself, it lost its status as a central prop of the bohemian experience. In serious fiction, drugs ceased to play much of a role as symbols of rebellion and individuality. To the extent that drugs figure at all in the American literature of the 1970s and 1980s, they are either glamorized by young writers who indulge themselves in an unseasoned flirtation with decadence, or portrayed as part and parcel of a desperate and despairing culture. Whatever happens next in the world of literature, one thing seems unthinkable, and that is that drugs will ever regain their allure as emblems of personal liberation.

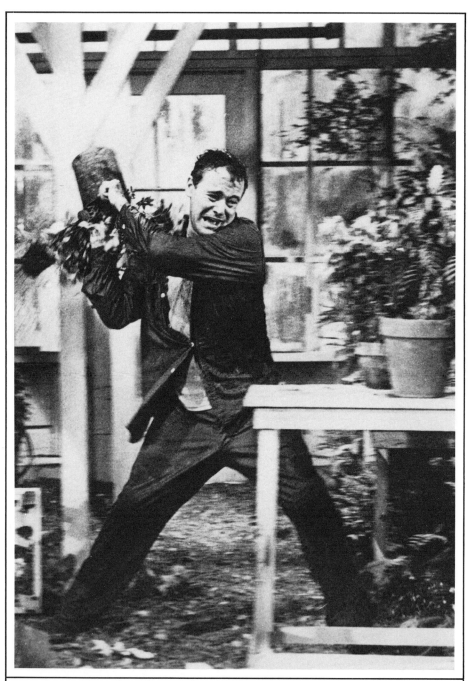

Jack Lemmon played an embattled alcoholic in the 1962 film Days of Wine and Roses. *The theme of drug abuse has figured prominently in many major productions of both stage and screen.*

CHAPTER 5

DRUGS ON THE STAGE AND SCREEN

The abuse of drugs has long been an important theme in the theater, from the temperance dramas of the 19th century to the harsh cynicism of contemporary plays. One of the first temperance dramas was the 1844 play *The Drunkard*. This production featured a straightforward plot concerning the fall of a decent family man through his abuse of alcohol, and his eventual return to goodness.

The Drunkard gave mid-19th-century audiences a sentimental morality play, but by the end of the 19th century playwrights in Europe and America began to hammer home messages with harsh realism.

One of these playwrights was a Russian named Aleksey Maksimovich Peshkov. Peshkov, who later changed his name to Maksim Gorky, had knocked around, hungry and homeless, doing odd jobs to survive, since he was a child. His compatriots were often the dregs of society, and he immortalized these anonymous men and women in his 1902 play *The Lower Depths*.

This drama takes place in a basement owned by a married couple who share their home with an alcoholic actor, a thief, an ex-convict, and some other down-and-out characters. There in the sunless cellar, they drink, dream, argue, and philosophize. An old tramp who has faith in the dignity of humankind visits them and tries to change their lives. The alcoholic actor stops drinking for a while, but later, after a series of violent episodes among the other characters, hangs himself.

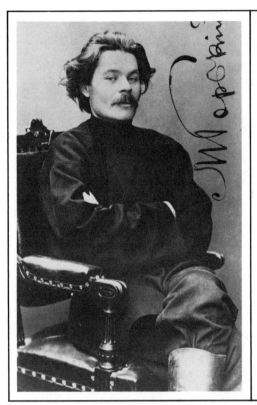

The Russian playwright Maksim Gorky immortalized many of his friends and compatriots in his classic play of alcoholism and destitution, The Lower Depths.

The plot of the *The Lower Depths* no doubt influenced the American playwright Eugene O'Neill, who in 1946 wrote a play similar in theme and story to Gorky's masterpiece. This play, *The Iceman Cometh*, describes the defeat and self-delusions of a group of boarders and regulars at Harry Hope's saloon-hotel, located in New York City. The aging men drown the realities of their failures with whiskey and lay their plans for success as they wait for Hickey, a salesman, to burst upon them with his boundless good cheer and free-spending ways.

When Hickey arrives, however, he announces that he has had the courage to face himself and lay his hopeless dreams to rest. He urges them to do the same. Hickey's action is like grabbing life preservers away from drowning men. His friends sink into a despair so deep not even whiskey seems to numb it.

Hickey admits that his wife Evelyn suffered for years with his drinking and infidelities, always forgiving him in the end. His answer to Evelyn's generous spirit was an uncontrollable hatred of her. He tells his friends that, before he came that day to the saloon, he shot his wife and then called the police. After the police take Hickey out of the bar, his friends console themselves with the belief that their old friend must be insane. They retreat once again to their dream world conjured out of a whiskey bottle.

Like Gorky's, O'Neill's early life was difficult, but the problems the latter had during childhood were due not to poverty but to his family. In fact, O'Neill turned his tortured relationship with his family into a Pulitzer Prize-winning play called *Long Day's Journey into Night*. Written in 1941 but not produced for the stage until 1956 — three years after the playwright's death — *Long Day's Journey into Night* is based on a day at the O'Neill family's summer home in New London, Connecticut.

The central tension in the play involves the father, James Tyrone, who is a washed-up actor, and his two sons, Jamie, an irresponsible roustabout, and Edmund, Jamie's sickly younger brother. The mother, Mary, is a quieter, pitiful pres-

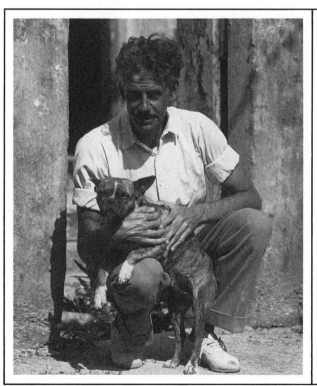

The plays of Eugene O'Neill were often autobiographical. One of his most famous plays, Long Day's Journey into Night, *is a tragedy that dramatizes the helplessness and despair of alcoholism and drug addiction.*

ence, having become a morphine addict years before at the hands of an incompetent physician. Lost in her private drug-induced world, Mary pathetically attempts to disguise her addiction. Much of the brutal dialogue among the men occurs during a long bout of drinking, at the end of which they simply sit and stare at each other as the final curtain falls.

O'Neill's plays are not just good theater; his work explores the psychology of drug abuse so relentlessly and realistically that both *Long Day's Journey into Night* and *The Iceman Cometh* have given modern physicians an insight into the problem.

A man's struggle to remain sober is depicted in William Inge's 1950 play *Come Back, Little Sheba*. The protagonist, Doc Delaney, has been a member of Alcoholics Anonymous for almost a year and is participating in the "Twelfth Step" stage of this program, which is the final phase of recovery. Tragically, failed opportunity, a passionless marriage, and repressed feelings of desire lure Doc back to alcohol. One night of drunkenness destroys Doc's recovery. He is once again a desperate man, shattered by alcohol.

A Product of Its Times

Not all dramas depict drug experiences as tragic and shattering. Indeed, the rock musical *Hair*, first performed off-Broadway in 1967 (on Broadway in 1968), boldly celebrated the use of psychoactive substances, a foolish and immature attitude toward drugs that was unfortunately rampant in the popular culture of the late 1960s and early 1970s. The play, which centers upon a group of young New York "hippies" opposed to war and supporting free love, devotes an entire scene to explaining the experience of an LSD "trip." This scene stresses the enhancement of visual aspects such as form and color that the drug can cause, while avoiding the negative aspects of LSD — the frightful hallucinations and feelings of paranoia that often occur in people under the influence of this substance.

Cynicism and Drugs

Dramas of the 1980s have brought back the grim reality of drug abuse. Cocaine, which has been used in epidemic proportions throughout the decade, is the substance of abuse in

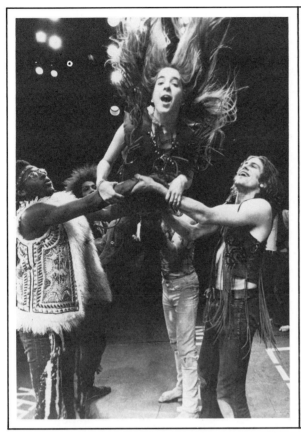

David Rabe's 1984 play *Hurlyburly*. The plot concerns four divorced men living in Hollywood who try to muscle their way through life with cynicism and drugs. For one character, Mickey, all emotional ties are temporary, and cocaine is an important means of sustenance. He says that he and his roommates are all "involved in a variety of pharmaceutical experiments," which as another character, Eddie, explains, "test the American dream of oblivion."

Hurlyburly differs significantly in its representation of drug use from the rest of the plays discussed in this chapter. Whereas plays such as *Long Day's Journey into Night*, *The Iceman Cometh*, and *Come Back, Little Sheba* present the tragic addictions of their characters in a largely sympathetic way, and *Hair* depicts an LSD trip as a glorious experience, *Hurlyburly* presents the abuse of cocaine as neither an affliction nor an adventure. It is simply a given in the fabric of its characters' daily lives.

Drugs and the Movies

Movies, too, have often reflected the horrors and sorrows of drug abuse. Indeed, the cinematic assault against alcohol began very early in movie history. Walter Haggar, a traveling moviemaker based in New South Wales, Australia, made *D.T.'s or the Effect of Drink* at the very beginning of the 20th century. As described in a 1905 catalogue issued by a British firm called the Gaumont Company, the movie recounts the story of a drunken young man's experience with the hallucinatory powers of alcohol. The catalogue's description, as summarized in *The History of the British Film, 1896–1908*, by Rachel Low and Roger Manvell, portrays the movie as an antidrinking film that is enlivened with humorous special effects.

The drunkard in the movie comes home and throws his coat onto a bed. The coat assumes the shape of a dog and walks away. The startled man then fights off a procession of bizarre creatures until, exhausted, he goes to bed. But as he flops down to sleep, the bed suddenly shifts to the other side of the room, leaving him lying on the floor.

The bed then turns into a monster that carries the drunkard around the room on its back. Finally, the bed disappears in a puff of smoke, catapulting the man into the sky. When he reaches earth again, the man vows that he will never again get drunk.

Alcohol: Crime and Disease

D.T.'s or the Effect of Drink certainly had an antialcohol theme, but it was done in a humorous, lighthearted way, with an "all's well that ends well" tone. Later movies portrayed alcohol and alcoholism far more darkly, reflecting the moralistic sentiments that lay behind Prohibition and even more importantly, a growing awareness of the real and terrible problem of chronic alcoholism.

Bootlegging was the theme in the 1931 movie *The Public Enemy*, which was made two years before Prohibition was repealed. The movie chronicles the rags-to-riches story of two poor Irish boys, Tom Powers (James Cagney) and Matt Doyle (Edward Woods), who turn first to petty theft and then to bootlegging to make their fortune. In fact, selling illegal liquor makes them very rich. Tom and Matt's luck runs

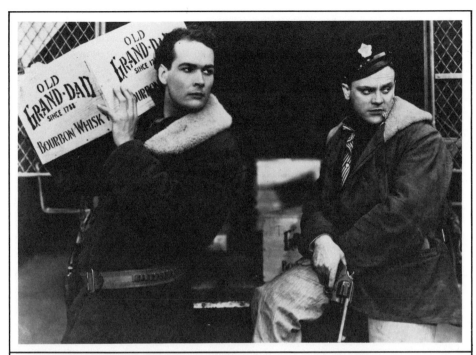

Edward Woods and James Cagney starred as two Irish boys who make their fortune as bootleggers in the 1931 film The Public Enemy.

out at the end of the film, however, when they are gunned down by other criminals involved in the illegal liquor rackets.

Fourteen years after *The Public Enemy*, Paramount Studios released a film exploring the misery of a chronic drinker. The movie, *The Lost Weekend*, depicts a few harrowing days in the life of Don Birnam (Ray Milland), a writer and alcoholic. Birnam is in the midst of an alcoholic binge, which results in his pawning his typewriter, stealing small amounts of cash, and attempting to take a woman's purse in order to raise money to support his drinking. A respite at Bellevue Hospital does little to help him, and in desperation he pawns his fiancée's coat to raise money for a gun to kill himself. Fortunately, the fiancée (played by Jane Wyman) talks him out of it, leaving the audience optimistic that he will recover.

Similar in theme to *The Lost Weekend* is the 1962 movie *Days of Wine and Roses*, which starred Jack Lemmon and Lee Remick as a husband and wife who fall victim to the horrors of alcohol addiction. Although the husband eventually gets help and is able to stop drinking, his wife is not quite so lucky and remains an alcoholic.

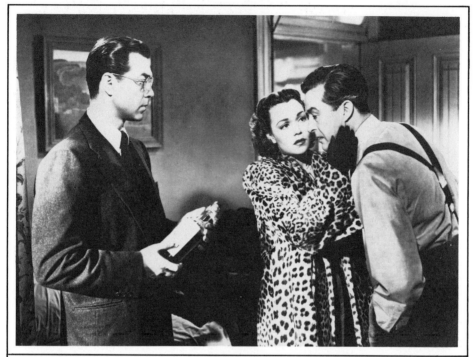

Jane Wyman comforts Ray Milland in a scene from the 1945 movie The Lost Weekend, *the saga of an alcoholic struggling to remain sober. Unlike many films about substance abuse, this drama ended happily.*

Human Wreckage: Morphine and Cocaine

Drugs other than alcohol have also had a long, colorful movie history. D. W. Griffith, the great moviemaker of the early years of film, made several movies about the evils of drink, including his last movie, *The Struggle* (1932). But in a 1911 movie, *For His Son*, Griffith took on the evils of cocaine with a story about an ambitious physician who invents a soft drink spiked with the drug. The doctor makes a great deal of money, but his son dies in his arms, one of the many victims of his father's concoction.

The antidrug campaign in movies took a particularly personal turn in 1923, after Wallace Reid, one of Hollywood's hot young stars, died of a morphine overdose while working on a movie set. Reid had become addicted to morphine after taking it to ease the pain of a leg injury sustained while making a movie. The studio bosses had continued to supply him with morphine, rather than lose his services while he kicked his habit in a sanitarium.

Reid's distraught wife, Dorothy Davenport, decided to spread the word about the dangers of narcotics. Her antidrug film, *Human Wreckage* (1923), was made with the cooperation of the Los Angeles Anti-Narcotic League. The movie opened with this foreword:

> Dope is the gravest menace which today confronts the United States. Immense quantities of morphine, heroin, and cocaine are yearly smuggled into America across the Canadian and Mexican borders. The dope ring is composed of rings within rings, the inner ring undoubtedly including men powerful in finance, politics and society. But the trail to the "men higher up" is cunningly covered. No investigator has penetrated the inner circle.

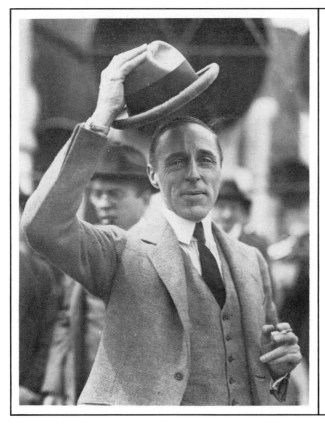

In 1911 D. W. Griffith, one of the great pioneers of film, made For His Son, *which was one of the first movies to tackle the theme of cocaine abuse.*

Reefer Madness

A decade later *Reefer Madness* (1936) debuted. It would become the classic antimarijuana film. The film now plays on college campuses, where it is considered a rather camp comedy because of its shrill message and melodramatic story, which involves a bunch of clean-cut men and women who become irreversibly corrupted when they start smoking marijuana.

Equally uncompromising in its depiction of drug addiction, but infinitely more realistic and powerful, Nelson Algren's novel *The Man with the Golden Arm* was turned into a harrowing movie in 1955. In the novel, the protagonist, a sharp-eyed poker dealer named Frankie Machine (played by Frank Sinatra in the movie), beats his heroin addiction while doing time in prison. He learns to play drums there, but before he is able to try out for a band on the outside after his release, Frankie is framed and sent back to prison. His old boss bails him out and in return wants Frankie to come back to deal one more game. Frankie goes back to the cards and back to the needle, and he ends up dying in a cheap hotel. (The ending of the movie is more upbeat: in an agonizingly realistic sequence Frankie kicks his heroin habit "cold turkey" with the support of his devoted girl friend, played by Kim Novak.)

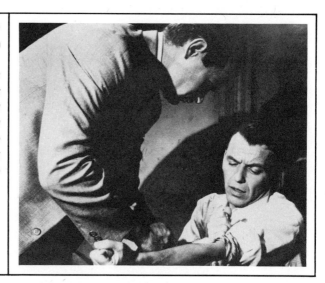

In this scene from the 1955 movie The Man with the Golden Arm, *one of Hollywood's more realistic treatments of drug abuse, recovering heroin addict Frankie Machine (Frank Sinatra) succumbs to temptation.*

Easy Rider

Epitomizing the attitude the entertainment community took toward drug use during the 1960s, *Easy Rider* (1969) presented it as an integral part of the rootless lifestyle of two young men (Dennis Hopper and Peter Fonda) who finance a trip across America by selling drugs. The movie features a long, rather disturbing scene in which the two travelers take LSD and hallucinate, and several segments in which the two men smoke marijuana; the entire movie is a sad, perhaps slightly and unintentionally ironic reflection of the decade's permissiveness regarding the use of drugs.

In 1971 Hollywood updated the nightmare world of junkies that had been so vividly portrayed in *The Man with the Golden Arm*. That year, *Panic in Needle Park* told the story of a young couple who share a hotel room and a heroin habit. Needle Park is the nickname for an area of Manhattan's Upper West Side that attracted junkies. The panic occurs when a shortage of heroin develops in the city.

Also that year, the drug genre took an even more realistic turn when real drug addicts starred in the explicitly detailed movie *Dusty and Sweets McGee*. As described by a reviewer for *The New York Times*, "The camera glues to a group of young and not-so-young junkies lolling and wallowing around Los Angeles. Their language, denoting an almost methodical drug addiction and most of it delivered in a paranoid whine or mumble, is filthy. The point, quite literally, is an interminable, almost loving focus on needle injections."

During this film one teenage boy ironically groans, "Life isn't all — — and dope. People do things." Later, he and his girl friend prepare an injection that accidentally kills him.

Drugs, the Law, and Hollywood

While *Dusty and Sweets McGee* was playing in Manhattan, the Knapp Commission was investigating corruption among the ranks of the New York City police. A young undercover officer, who lived in Greenwich Village and often dressed like a hippie, testified against fellow officers who were accepting bribes from criminals, including drug dealers. The scandal shook the police department. The young detective, Frank Serpico, suffered a head wound during a drug bust and eventually resigned and moved to Switzerland. His story, presented in the book *Serpico*, was made into the 1973 movie of the same name.

Drug smuggling provided the theme for *The French Connection* (1971), an account of how law enforcement officials busted up an international heroin smuggling ring. The film turned a New York City police detective who worked on that case into a movie star. Detective Eddie Eagan (portrayed as Popeye Doyle by Gene Hackman in the movie) and his partner, Detective Salvatore Grosso, had discovered a multi-million-dollar stash of heroin hidden in the car of a French television personality. Starting with that evidence, the detectives unraveled a network of criminals bringing heroin into the United States.

Eagan had a role as a policeman in *The French Connection* (which had formerly been a book) and later starred in other movies and television programs. In *The French Connection* the ringleader escapes, although others in the ring are captured or killed. In *The French Connection II* (1975), Doyle kills him. (Christian Jacques David, the French citizen sentenced to 20 years in prison for heading up the real-life ring, was actually released from federal prison in 1985, seven years early, for good behavior.)

The 1980s

The 1982 film *I'm Dancing as Fast as I Can*, which was based on the 1972 book by television producer Barbara Gordon, took a serious look at a growing problem among adults: addiction to tranquilizers. The film is, in fact, an autobiography of Gordon, who became dependent on Valium and suffered devastating withdrawal effects when she attempted to stop taking the tranquilizer.

Drawing on a bygone era, the 1983 movie *Eddie and the Cruisers*, which recounts the rise to prominence of a 1960s rock group, borrows heavily from the life of Rimbaud for its storyline. The band's lyricist, who is an avid reader of Rimbaud's work, introduces the band's female singer to Rimbaud's semiautobiographical poem, "A Season in Hell."

At the end of the movie, the band's leader, Eddie, becomes enraged when he can not get his group's latest album recorded. The music in the album, which is titled *A Season in Hell*, is apparently ahead of its time and not commercial enough. In disgust, Eddie suddenly drops from sight, as Rim-

The 1973 film Serpico, *which was based on a true story, starred Al Pacino as a detective who testified against his fellow police officers for accepting bribes — including illicit substances — from criminals.*

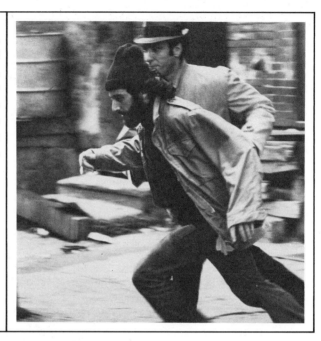

baud did, and the band breaks up. The music to this movie became quite popular, and one song, which was the title song of the group's ill-fated album, was titled *A Season in Hell*.

Another autobiographical film, *Jo Jo Dancer, Your Life Is Calling* (1986), traced the life and times of comedian Richard Pryor, who accidentally set himself on fire while preparing cocaine by a method called freebasing and almost died from his burns. Pryor, who starred as Jo Jo Dancer in the movie, was addicted to cocaine at the time and later kicked the habit.

By the 1980s, then, films and theatrical productions alike had moved, in their representations of drug use, from lurid and sensational excess — as in, for example, the movie *Reefer Madness* — to sometimes sensible, sometimes cynical, sometimes decadent, sometimes flippant realism. When they turn their attention to drug use, what cinematic and dramatic artists are telling us about drugs is a rough approximation of reality: sagas of wasted lives, destruction of families, crime, cruelty, corruption, and death. The romanticizing impulse with regard to drugs is all but dead. Plays and films now reflect the actual effects of drugs on society, and for the most part, those effects are grim.

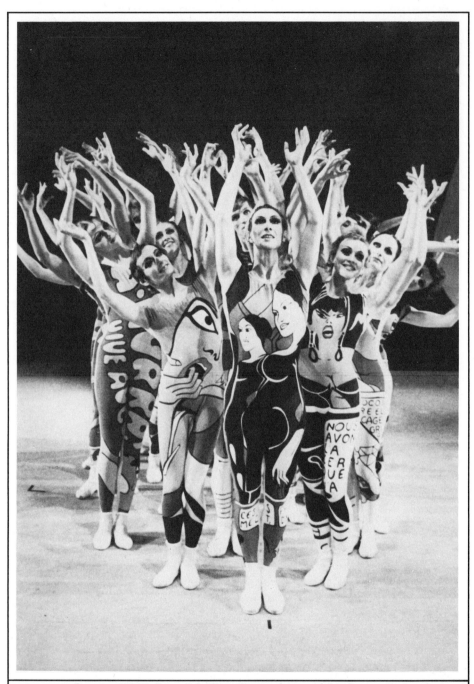

A scene from a 1971 "pop" ballet. Drugs have played a varied role in dance throughout the ages, from the wine-induced rituals of the ancient world to the publicized addictions of modern ballet stars.

CHAPTER 6

DRUGS AND DANCE

The art of dancing stands at the source of all the arts that express themselves first in the human person. . . . If we are indifferent to the art of dancing, we have failed to understand, not merely the supreme manifestation of physical life, but also the supreme symbol of spiritual life.

—Havelock Ellis
The Dance of Life, 1923

The art of dancing as a means of expressing emotion or narrating a story emerged very early in the existence of humankind. The religious aspects of dance also go back to ancient culture, and are often connected to, and indeed influenced by, drugs.

Drugs and Dance in Primitive Cultures

The mixing of drugs and dance for religious purposes is a characteristic of some ceremonies in primitive societies and goes back as far as 10,000 years. In these religions or cults the religious official, the shaman, goes into a trance and becomes possessed by a spirit, who works through the shaman. Shamanism still exists in the arctic and central Asian regions,

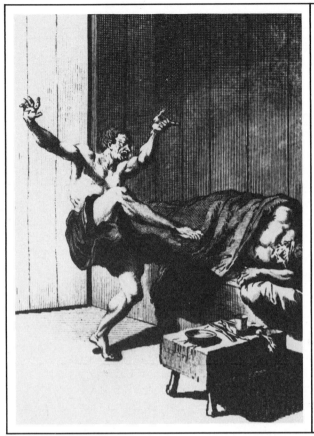

A shaman exorcises a sick man's demon. Some tribal religions believe that shamans, or medicine men, can, through the performance of an opium-induced dance, conjure up spirits that cure illness.

Southeast Asia, Oceania, and among many South and North American aboriginal tribes. The shaman is a medicine man/priest who cures sickness, escorts the soul of the dead to the other world, or cleanses the body of evil spirits. He does this by attaining a state of ecstasy through dancing, music, contemplation, and, sometimes, the ingestion of hallucinogens.

Shamans of Southeast Asia often use opium to increase the ecstatic effects of dancing, through which their spirits soar up into the supernatural realm, where they receive the power to cure illness or divine the future.

In Fiji, ceremonial dancers perform during the preparation of a sacred drink called kava (also spelled cava or ava). Fijians drink this beverage, which is made from the pepper plant, principally *Piper methysticum*, during the kava ceremony. Although it is nonalcoholic, an active ingredient renders the concoction intoxicating: the drink is used as a narcotic for its relaxing effect.

The Ancient Greeks and Romans

In ancient Greece, drinking and dancing were an integral part of the rites that celebrated Dionysus, the Greek god of wine. The religion of Dionysus began at least as far back as the 6th century B.C.E., probably in Thrace (now part of Greece and Bulgaria) and Phrygia (now part of Turkey).

During the Dionysian rites, female attendants, called bacchantes or maenads, became possessed with the spirit of the god through music, dancing, and liberal doses of wine. They indulged in orgiastic meals, during which they tore apart animals with their bare hands and devoured the meat. The wild and frenzied joy experienced by the women took place originally in secret, away from men. Only later, apparently, did the rite evolve into a revelry that included males, and presumably at least some promiscuity. Euripides, the famous 5th-century B.C.E. Greek poet, wrote of these goings-on in his drama *The Bacchantes*.

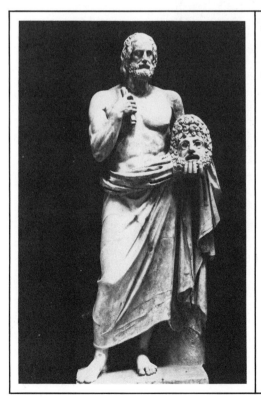

Euripides, one of the foremost tragedians of ancient Greece, incorporated the drunken dance and revelry of the Dionysian rites in his play The Bacchantes, *the last great Greek tragedy.*

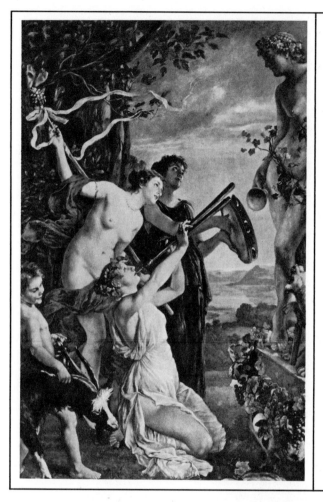

The Adoration of Dionysus, *by C.A. Geiger. In classical Athens, Dionysus, god of wine, was honored twice every year in elaborate festivals that involved heavy alcohol consumption and joyous dancing.*

Dionysian rites eventually evolved into a ritual during which a priest sang of life, death, and Dionysus, while the participants danced. In this fashion, the ancient, private celebrations of female followers of Dionysus led to the development of the dithyramb — a form of choral lyric with exchanges between the leader and the chorus — and ultimately to the development of Greek theater and theater dance. (Long after the actual movements were forgotten, the famous 20th-century American dancer Isadora Duncan—who often wore a Greek tunic — and the British dancer Ruby Ginner attempted to revive Greek dance theater in the United States and Great Britain respectively.)

The Greek rites were transplanted to ancient Rome. But the stolid Romans, taken aback by the bacchanalia, as these ancient drinking and dancing rites were called there, passed a decree in 186 B.C.E. prohibiting them throughout the region now known as Italy. Nevertheless, bacchanalias continued for many years.

Danse Macabre

After the fall of the Roman Empire, theatrical dance disappeared. But during the medieval period, in addition to whatever dance revelry existed among the common folk, the dance of death (or in French, *danse macabre*) emerged as an allegorical device in the drama, poetry, music, and visual arts of western Europe.

Reflecting the waves of mass death caused by plagues and wars, this dance consisted of a procession or dance of living figures following the image of death, often to the grave.

The practice of the dance of death became less common during the Renaissance, a period that nurtured the reemergence of the arts, including dancing, in Italy. But dancing ran afoul of the strict doctrines of the Puritan movement in England which started around the mid-1500s. In fact, the Puritans linked the social activities of drinking and dancing, and they discouraged dancing in an attempt to regulate morality. Unfortunately, prohibiting dancing did not decrease the consumption of alcohol during this period — rather, it had the opposite effect.

In his 1923 book *The Dance of Life*, Havelock Ellis denounced the discouragement of dance by the Puritans of 400 years before and quoted the French writer Rémy de Gourmont's remark about the evil that took the place of dance: "The drinking shop conquered the dance, and alcohol replaced the violin."

The Birth of Ballet

While Puritanism was stifling dance in England during the 16th century, a new form of dance was maturing in France. Originating in Italy before the 16th century, this new dance combined movement, music, decor, and special effects. The first example of this dance form was presented at the French court of Catherine de Médicis in 1581. This production, *Le Ballet comique de la reine*, was the ancestor of modern ballet.

It was not until the 18th century, however, that the virtuoso dancer Marie Camargo gained greater freedom of movement by shortening the length of her skirt. Ballet as an art form did not see many innovations in the early and mid-19th century but underwent a renaissance in Russia after 1875. The Russian ballet dancers trained more rigorously than any had before, and Russian ballet has been maintained at the highest level of professionalism ever since.

The Contemporary Scene

The rigorous physical demands made on modern ballet dancers have often driven them to control their weight through the use of amphetamines and over-the-counter diet pills. Alcohol is also a problem; the pressures of ballet make it difficult for some dancers to avoid alcohol. In his autobiographical book, *Leap Year*, ballet dancer Christopher d'Amboise admits that at one point during the year of his life portrayed in the book, he found "the most enjoyable part of the day is the end of it, when I can return home and sit in bed with my feet propped up and a six-pack of beer in my lap.... Each morning I am disgusted at the sight of six empty bottles; each night I open six more."

Isadora Duncan, the innovative American modern dancer, also used alcohol. Having heard that some Russians started drinking vodka in the morning to cure their hangovers, she flirted with the idea of substituting vodka for her morning coffee; there is no reason to believe, though, that this was anything more than a passing affectation.

In 1967, two other masters of the art, Dame Margot Fonteyn and Rudolf Nureyev of Britain's Royal Ballet, found themselves in the middle of a small drug scandal. The two dancers made news when police arrested them at a house party in the Haight-Ashbury district of San Francisco, the stomping ground of the city's large hippie population. Angered by the raucous crowd and the blaring music, neighbors had called the police, who raided the house, found marijuana cigarettes on the premises, and arrested everyone they could collar. A news story reported that police found Nureyev sprawled face down on the roof of the building, and Dame Margot, in her mink coat, crouched behind a low wall nearby.

Nureyev and Fonteyn were released immediately, and the charges were dropped. In her 1976 book, *Margot Fon-*

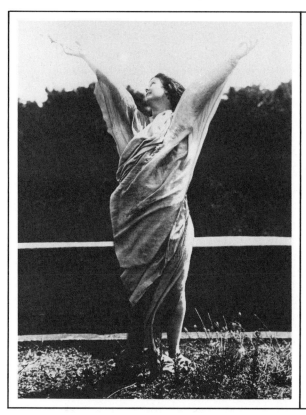

Although Isadora Duncan, the unconventional pioneer of modern dance in the United States, experimented with alcohol for a brief time, there is no evidence that she used psychoactive drugs regularly.

teyn: Autobiography, Fonteyn claimed that she was an innocent bystander. Back in England a reporter asked Dame Margot's mother if her daughter might actually have been smoking marijuana. She replied, "How can you dance if you take drugs?"

That question received a dramatic answer in 1984 when Gelsey Kirkland, a former American Ballet Theatre principal, left the company after her erratic behavior and unreliability disrupted her career. Later, in her autobiography, *Dancing on My Grave*, she detailed the reason for her problem: cocaine addiction. According to the book, cocaine use is not uncommon in the world of ballet.

After successfully fighting her problem and working to regain her form, Kirkland appeared for the first time in two years at the Royal Opera House at Covent Garden, England, on April 11, 1986. She had kicked the habit and returned to rave reviews.

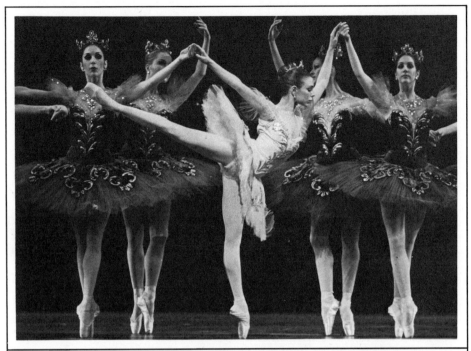

In her 1986 autobiography, Dancing on My Grave, *Gelsey Kirkland* revealed that she had been dependent on cocaine. Kirkland overcame her addiction and returned to the stage in 1986.

In 1981 *Dance Magazine* ran a series of articles describing the conditions leading to the increase of drug abuse problems in the United States, pointing out that drugs of abuse have become easily accessible; that in our society we have been conditioned to seek instant solutions to pain and stress and turn, however misguidedly, to drugs for this reason; and that drug use is widely accepted in many social circles.

The series also offered advice to dancers on how to deal with personal and professional pressures without resorting to drugs, as well as how to respond to the arguments of fellow artists who look to drugs as the answer to fatigue, sleeplessness, anxiety, or depression.

Another way the profession has responded to the scourge of drug abuse among performing artists is the establishment of special medical programs. One such program is the Performing Arts Center for Health (PACH) in New York City. Included in this medical service is access to psychiatric counseling at New York University Medical Center/Bellevue Hospital. This part of the service responds to all psychiatric needs, including drug abuse.

Efforts such as this would probably have won the hearty approval of writer and dance devotee Havelock Ellis, who regarded dancing as a pure, primal art and "the loftiest, the most moving, the most beautiful of the arts, because it is no mere translation of abstraction from life; it is life itself."

The abuse of one's life through drugs, then, would seem only to jeopardize the artistic purity of the creative impulse that initially motivates the dancer.

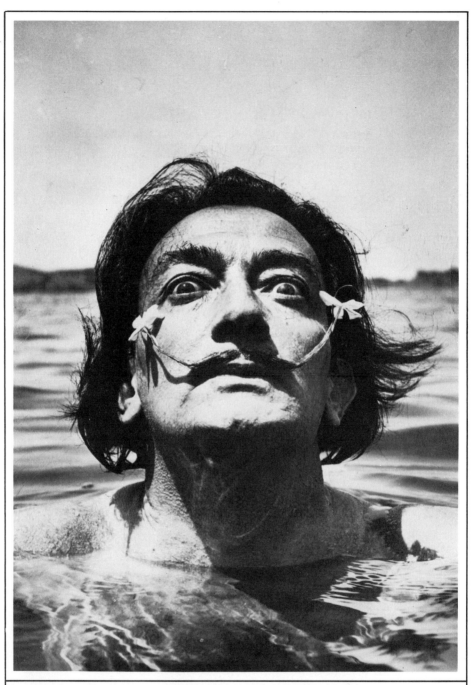

The paintings of the great surrealist artist Salvador Dali represent hallucinatory landscapes in which disjointed images combine to evoke the unreality of a dream world.

CHAPTER 7

DRUGS, PAINTING, AND SCULPTURE

The god Dionysus reclines on the deck of an ancient ship plying the waters toward Greece. A grapevine laden with the divine fruit spirals up around the ship's mast, and dolphins frolic in the water.

This scene, painted on the inside of a shallow Greek bowl about 540 B.C.E., illustrates a story in which Dionysus was abducted by pirates. But when he caused grapevines to grow all over the ship, frightening his captors, they jumped overboard and were turned into dolphins. This event was celebrated by the Greeks, a testament to their love for Dionysus, the god of wine.

As we have seen, Dionysus founded an ancient, mysterious cult of women — joined eventually by men — who worshiped him. Their rites of Dionysus have been preserved by painters and sculptors through the ages.

Ironically, it was the Romans, who had adopted the cult from the Greeks but banned it in 186 B.C.E., who succeeded in preserving for modern scholars the only wall paintings that graphically disclose some of those rites.

About 50 B.C.E., a talented but unknown painter created a colorful frieze now titled *Scenes of a Dionysiac Mystery Cult* in the Villa of the Mysteries just outside Pompeii, which was an ancient town near what is now the city of Naples,

Italy. The artist placed figures of the cult's men and women on a ledge of green set against a pattern of red panels that are separated by strips of black. The cult members enact their rituals upon this series of stages. In one scene, for example, a girl undergoes a whipping as part of her initiation into the Dionysian mysteries. In another scene a seated, bearded man offers a jug of wine to a young male initiate, while another man holds up a horrible mask behind him.

The Legacy of Dionysus

The legacy of Dionysus and his Roman counterpart, Bacchus, survived the decision of the 4th-century emperor Constantine the Great to legalize Christianity in the Roman Empire,

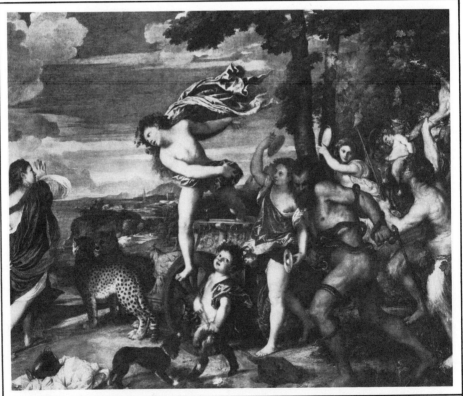

Bacchus and Ariadne, *by the Venetian Renaissance painter Titian. Abandoned by her former love, Theseus, and in deep despair, Ariadne recoils in fear from the god of wine.*

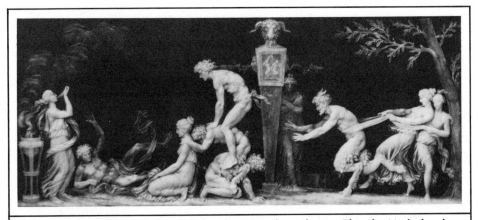

Nymphs and Satyrs, *a relief by the French sculptor Claude Michel, also known as Clodion. In Greek mythology the satyrs were attendants of Dionysus and indulged freely in lecherous and wild revelry.*

thus aiding the growth of that religion at the expense of paganism. The tradition of classic Greek and Roman sculpture was, in fact, influential long after Constantine's death, giving rise to such "classical" works as *Priestess of Bacchus*, an ivory-carved leaf forming the right half of a diptych (hinged pair of paintings or carvings) produced about 390–400 C.E.

Thousands of years later, the great Renaissance painter Titian, who became the finest painter in Venice, produced paintings based on the myths of Bacchus. Titian's *Bacchanal* (1518), certainly a pagan work of art, is populated with joyous, healthy young men and women dancing, reclining, and drinking in an otherwise serene, bucolic clearing.

A few years later, still influenced by myths of the ancient god, Titian painted *Bacchus and Ariadne* (1523). It is a scene from one of the tales of the life of Bacchus and his wife, Ariadne, whom he wed after she was abandoned by her former love, Theseus. In Titian's rendition, Bacchus is suspended in midair as he approaches Ariadne, while a group of merrymakers press forward from the woods.

The cult of Dionysus continued to influence artists into the 18th century. About a year before the beginning of the American Revolution, the French sculptor Claude Michel, who called himself Clodion, created his terra cotta (hardbaked pottery) sculpture *Satyr and Bacchante*, a sexually suggestive study of a pair of Dionysian celebrants.

The Rake's Progress

In the 18th century, classical revelry gave way to outright orgy when the English painter William Hogarth began to produce his "morality plays." These plays were actually unified sets of pictures. Scene III of one of these sets, *The Rake's Progress*, is a riotous rendition of a young man's overindulgence in wine and women. Titled *The Orgy*, it shows a room full of men and women surrounding a table. Two of the women attend to the foppishly dressed young rake, who is resting his right foot on the table as one of the women loosens the top of his shirt.

Hogarth also did engravings, one of which, *Gin Lane* (1751), depicted alcohol abuse by the lower classes of London, a problem that had reached epidemic proportions.

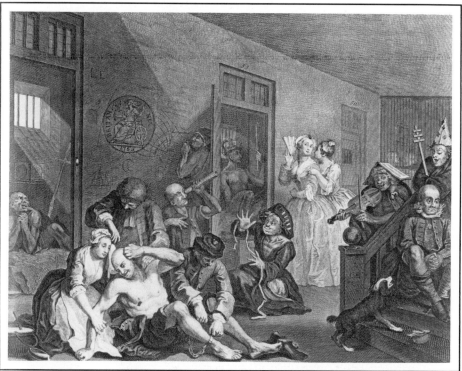

The 18th-century English artist William Hogarth's The Rake's Progress *combines a moral tale of a young man's overindulgence in wine and women with harsh depictions of contemporary social conditions.*

Experiments and Discoveries

Less than a hundred years after *The Rake's Progress*, the boisterous consumption of alcohol in France spread from the artists' studios to the bars, where advocates of a new school of French painting held court, drinking, arguing, and condemning their artistic adversaries.

The heated debate took place between artists of the older, classical style of painting supported by the extremely influential French Academy of Fine Arts (which controlled much of the teaching and government purchases of art; its members served on the juries that chose paintings for the biennial art shows, called salons), and the newer, radical painters who incorporated novel techniques into their works.

This was the mid-19th century, the height of the Romantic movement, which, as mentioned in Chapter 2, was a time of experimentation. It was an age when authors, artists, philosophers, and scientists were exploring new ideas and making exciting discoveries.

The artistic revolt burning within the radical painters of this period had been inspired by recent scientific theories on light and the response of the human eye to it. Of major importance was the discovery by Eugène Chevreul of the phenomenon called "negative afterimage." Chevreul showed that a color seen alone seems to be surrounded by a faint halo of its complementary color, that is, its color of maximum contrast. (The phenomenon can easily be experienced by staring at a red dot against a white surface for 30 to 60 seconds before shifting the eye to stare at a blank white surface. A light, greenish afterimage will briefly be seen. Green is complementary to red.)

Claude Monet incorporated such discoveries into his 1874 painting *Impression: Sunrise*. A hostile critic's jibes at this departure from realism gave birth to the term "Impressionism." The Impressionist artists juxtaposed colors in their paintings for the eye to fuse together at a distance; the painters also tinged shadows with colors complementary to the object casting the shadow. In addition, they sometimes painted landscapes devoid of people.

Outraged at this violation of classical form, the French Academy of Fine Arts, which emphasized clear outlines and sharp contrasts of light and shade (and landscapes populated

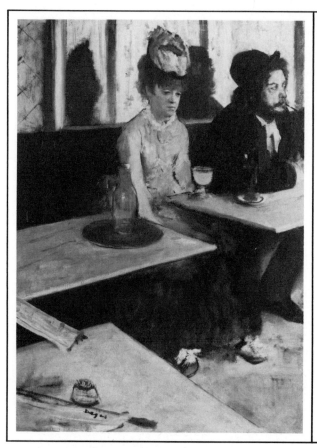

L'Absinthe, *a painting by the Impressionist artist Edgar Degas, epitomizes the sense of alienation and estrangement that haunts alcoholics and other drug abusers.*

with noble, idealized figures), refused to display Impressionist paintings at the salons. This only added fuel to the fire of debate and hardened positions on both sides.

A group of Impressionists, including Monet, Edouard Manet, and Edgar Degas, gathered regularly at the Café Guerbois in Paris, where, amid discussions, arguments, and downright quarrelsome exchanges, they learned from each other and kept one another's "wits sharpened," as Monet later recalled. These meetings also served to rally the cause against the art establishment. Not surprisingly, these drinking establishments began to figure prominently in the work produced by Impressionists. Manet even composed a pen-and-ink drawing of a scene of himself at the Café Guerbois.

Degas used another Parisian bar, Café de la Nouvelle-Athènes, as a backdrop for his 1876 painting *L'Absinthe*, a study of the brooding loneliness of a couple sitting at a table in an empty corner of this bar. The woman sits staring, disenchanted, with a glass of absinthe on the table in front of her. Because absinthe was highly toxic, it was eventually banned in most Western countries early in the 20th century.

Edouard Manet's last major painting, *A Bar at the Folies-Bergère*, completed in 1882, contrasts the figure of a melancholy barmaid with the image of the gaiety of its patrons, reflected in the large mirror behind her. This work is more famous for its disturbing mirror imagery and peculiar dimensions than for its subject matter. However, the fact that Manet chose a café for his setting is indicative of the popularity of bars as a gathering place for the 19th-century Parisian bourgeoisie, the class of people Manet chose to portray.

Drinking was not confined to nighttime gatherings at bars, however. During this period France was a world of

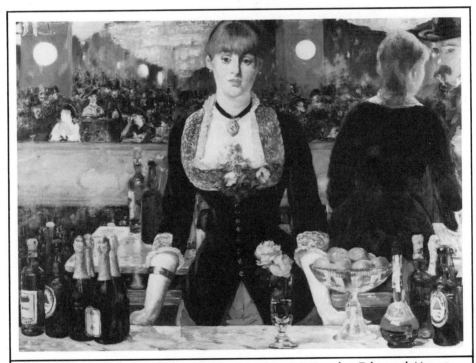

A Bar at the Folies-Bergère, the last major painting by Edouard Manet, depicts through a mirror image life in a Parisian cafe. Bars were popular gathering places for the 19th-century French bourgeoisie.

picnics, boating parties, and outdoor cafés. The people who could manage to enjoy life did so. Another Impressionist painter, Auguste Renoir, captured this spirit of eat, drink, and be merry in *La Moulin de la falette*, an animated portrait of people gathering to drink, eat, and socialize outdoors.

Decadence and Nihilism

Even as such romantic Impressionist visions were being put onto canvas, the dark clouds of another age were gathering. The decadent age of the late 19th and early 20th centuries suffused the literary and artistic climate with feelings of nihilism. Arthur Rimbaud's idea of deranging the senses was in some ways, perhaps, the literary equivalent of life in the Pa-

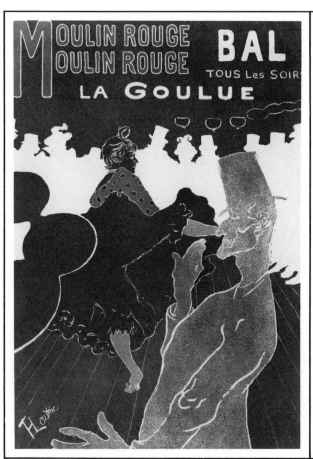

At The Moulin Rouge, a poster by the 19th-century artist Henri de Toulouse-Lautrec, who was a habitué of this Parisian cabaret and other night spots.

risian fast lane during the late 1800s. And perhaps no artist represents this after-hours world better than Henri de Toulouse-Lautrec.

Born in 1864 in Albi, France, Toulouse-Lautrec moved to Paris to study painting at the age of 18, eventually settling in the section called Montmartre. Here he enjoyed the night-life of Paris, especially the raucous dance halls.

Perhaps Toulouse-Lautrec's exaggerated life of gaiety was his escape from the pain of his disfigurement; dwarflike, he had out-turned lips, a bulbous nose, and tiny legs. People on the street made fun of him as he shuffled by in his baggy clothes and bowler hat.

His raucous lifestyle conflicted with that of his rather serious friend, Vincent van Gogh, with whom he occasionally lingered over glasses of absinthe. It might have been during one of these conversations with van Gogh that Toulouse-Lautrec discussed his fascination with portraying drunkenness. Drawing on discussions with van Gogh, and inspired by the painting *L'Absinthe* by his hero Degas, Toulouse-Lautrec painted his great study of intoxication, *Drunkard;* or *The Tippler*, in 1889. He had a genius for rendering the pain of alcoholism, and he portrayed his subjects pitilessly.

One of his most famous works, *At the Moulin Rouge* (1892), portrays a famous Parisian dance hall he enjoyed visiting and the people who patronized it. Seated at a table in the middle of the picture are several of his friends, including Maurice Guibert, a representative of a famous champagne company who encouraged the painter to indulge his weakness for alcohol. The painter put himself into the picture as well: a short figure of a man walking alongside a much taller man in the background.

Toulouse-Lautrec, a bright light of the frivolous, frenetic nightlife of Montmartre, became an alcoholic. Although he did at one time abstain from the drug, he died from alcoholism in 1901, just before his 37th birthday.

One of Toulouse-Lautrec's friends was an attractive and ambitious young model named Suzanne Valadon. Her son Maurice, who was adopted by the writer Miguel Utrillo, also turned to painting. Like his mother's friend Toulouse-Lautrec, Utrillo's favorite scenes were of Paris, especially Montmartre. Like his mother's friend, he became an alcoholic and the disease stripped him of much of his artistic power.

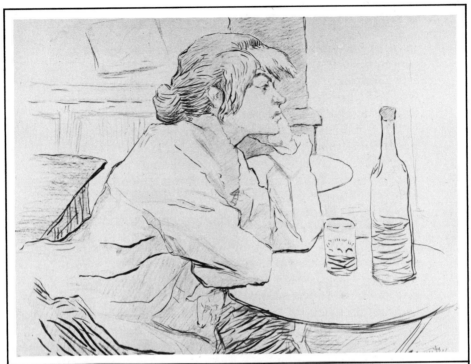

The Drunkard is a more serious work by Toulouse-Lautrec. Himself an alcoholic, this artist often portrayed drunkenness in his works.

The influence of alcohol on art has continued into the 20th century. Of particular interest is one of the Cubist works by Pablo Picasso. Cubism fragmented and redefined objects from several views simultaneously, a far cry from the romantic vibrancy of Impressionism. Yet this radical French school of art is called to mind in Picasso's Cubist sculpture *Glass of Absinthe*, a bronze structure painted in decorative patterns, to which a silver spoon is attached.

Although the surrealistic movement begun in Paris around 1924 had its representatives in the literary world, it was a deeply animating force on the visual arts as well. As we have said, surrealism had its roots in the French poets such as Baudelaire and Rimbaud, and the Italian painter Giorgio de Chirico; it emphasized expression of imagination as disclosed in dreams. One of the most prominent surrealist artists, Salvador Dali, produced the sexually suggestive work *Aphrodisiac Jacket*. For this piece he decorated a tuxedo with shot glasses filled with the liqueur crème de menthe, above a hanger to which a brassiere ad was attached.

Opium Myths and the Imagination

The predominance of alcohol over marijuana in Western art probably reflects the relatively late arrival of the drug-producing species of cannabis from the East, where it had been used for thousands of years. As we pointed out in Chapter 1, the ancient religious books of India — the *Vedas* — contain references to marijuana. The art of the region, likewise, had for many centuries included images of people using marijuana. Paintings and manuscript illustrations from at least the 14th century portray the use of this drug.

According to Alethea Hayter's *Opium and the Romantic Imagination*, the great German Renaissance artist Albrecht Dürer unwittingly created a lifelike image of "the peculiar

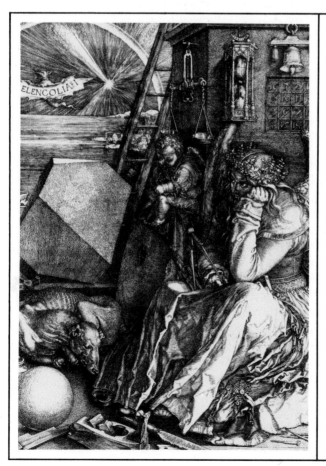

Melancholia, *by the German Renaissance artist Albrecht Dürer. There is no evidence to suggest that Dürer ever used psychoactive substances; the figure in this engraving, however, has come to symbolize for many the depression and despair of the drug addict.*

wretchedness of the drug addict" in his 1514 engraving titled *Melancholia*. The figure, a powerful winged female form, sits in a hunched, contemplative pose, a compass in her right hand opened for measuring, with various symbolic items in the background, such as a stone polyhedron (a many-sided object) and a pot on the fire.

Opium addiction, a scourge of several of the Romantic writers of the 19th century, was also graphically portrayed by artists of that time. When Baudelaire translated Edgar Allan Poe's book *Tales*, the frontispiece was adorned with an engraving of a brooding, seated woman holding a compass and an empty goblet, gazing downward toward the left side of the picture — an image based on Dürer's *Melancholia* but associated with the opium myths of both Poe and Baudelaire.

A further evolution of Dürer's engraving is Eugene Grasset's lithograph *Drug Addict*, which shows a seated, dark-haired young woman staring down toward the left of the picture. The pointed needle of the compass has evolved here into the needle of a hypodermic syringe, with which the woman is injecting herself in her leg.

Psychedelics and Hallucinogens

Psychedelic drugs, too, played a role in art long before the term was popularized by Timothy Leary, the Harvard professor who urged the youth of the 1960s to "tune in, turn on, and drop out," and was himself a heavy experimenter with LSD. The so-called magic mushroom, which contains the hallucinogenic compounds psilocybin and psilocin, appears to have influenced the art of the ancient Aztecs.

In their book *Psychedelic Art*, Robert E. L. Masters and Jean Houston point out that stone sculptures from the Guatemalan highlands dating as far back as 1500 B.C.E. portray mushrooms with the head of a god emerging from the stem. The authors also point out that Aztec art predating the Spanish conquest of Mexico in the 1520s shows the goddess of the sacred (psychedelic) mushroom using that plant to tempt the god Quetzalcoatl.

Native American Art

Drugs appear to have had a long history of influencing art in the United States as well.

In 1976 a New York pathologist, Klaus Wellmann, published a report in the *Journal of the American Medical Association*, in which he stated that some of the finest rock paintings of the early American Indians might have been created while the artists were under the influence of hallucinogenic drugs, which they had taken for ceremonial purposes.

According to Wellmann, the designs of cave artists of the Chumash and Yokuts Indians in California, and people living in the lower Pecos River region of Texas prior to the 1st century C.E., appeared to depict multicolored designs similar to those visualized in drug-induced trances.

Wellmann also pointed out that jimsonweed plants, which contain the vision-inducing alkaloids scopolamine and atropine, grew near the Chumash and Yokuts' caves. The Indians concocted a hallucinogenic drink by grinding the plant's roots, stems, and leaves, then soaking them in water.

The Chumash apparently regarded one particular species of jimsonweed as the source of all supernatural power. Under its influence, according to Wellmann, the Indians visualized birds, animals, and supernatural beings.

One of the first plants containing "magic" drugs discovered by Indians in the American Southwest was *Lophophora williamsii*, a spherical cactus (mescal button) containing a drug called peyote, whose active substance is mescaline, a powerful hallucinogenic drug chemically related to the neurotransmitter dopamine.

Some of the 20th-century Native American artists who have incorporated peyote-influenced visions are Ernest Spybuck, Stephen Mopope, and Tsa Toke. Tsa Toke, who was a Kiowa Indian, died in 1956. The Kiowas had settled in the central plains area of the United States by 1500 C.E. Toke painted mystical visions of the peyote cactus, impressions of the nightlong religious ceremony of the Native American Church called the peyote ritual, and symbols that he first saw as hallucinogenic images.

In *Psychedelic Art* Masters and Houston quote Toke, who wrote of one of his psychedelic experiences:

> I went into a meeting once and had a vision. I took the herb once and began to understand the time had come for further knowledge about this Cormorant Bird. The consciousness awakened.

Toke afterward used the cormorant as a religious symbol in much of his art.

Such Indian art is much more formalized than many of the free-flowing patterns and colors of later, non-Indian psychedelic art. Toke's *Morning in Peyote Tepee* is an example of this formalized imagery. It depicts a group of Indians seated in a circle inside a tepee that is flanked by religious images. Stephen Mopope's watercolor *Peyote Meeting* uses somewhat similar imagery in depicting the peyote ceremony.

LSD and Creativity

The psychedelic drug LSD made its mark on both society and art during the 1960s and 1970s. In 1969 Richard Hartmann, a German psychiatrist and art dealer working in conjunction with the Max Planck Institute for Psychiatry, tested the effects of the drug on the creativity of 34 artists. A record of the experiment, shown on West German television in December of that year, was titled *The Artificial Paradises*, presumably after Baudelaire's two-part book on the effects of hashish and opium.

Artists with a variety of styles were given LSD and directed their attention to their craft. According to a news account of the experiment, most of the artists discovered that they could not concentrate on their work, as images poured out of their subconscious in rapid succession. One artist, Bernhard Jager, complained that he could not draw because "everything begins to move on this picture. The ears of a wolf turn into a burning pine forest."

Almost all the artists experienced a temporary decline in their skills. Dr. Hartmann concluded that for creative artists, the drug was more likely to produce negative than positive effects on their creativity.

Nevertheless, "psychedelic art," as it was called, burst onto the scene during the 1960s as awareness of LSD's mind-altering properties became more common. Eastern religions became associated with LSD "trips," and the Oriental mandala, a circular, concentric arrangement of geometric shapes representing the cosmos, became incorporated into this new form of art.

In "head shops" (establishments where drug paraphernalia is sold) catering to hippie clientele, mandala prints hung on walls and various psychedelic designs swirled about on

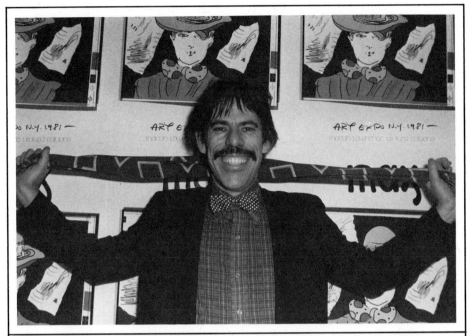

The works of Peter Max, which were extremely popular in the 1960s, captured the hallucinatory visions induced by drugs such as mescaline and LSD and helped make psychedelic art commercially acceptable.

both posters and postcards. Artist Peter Max produced popular psychedelic poster art and was commissioned to do a variety of commercial works during the late 1960s and early 1970s.

But psychedelic art was more than trivial experiments and poster art. Artists who took LSD and other hallucinogens during the 1960s used their experience to produce elaborate, thoughtful work. The drugs did not give them the ability to create art. The artists had to use the raw materials of their own intelligence, imagination, and talent to incorporate this new experience into the images they put on canvas.

Among the serious psychedelic artists were Isaac Abrams, Arlene Sklar-Weinstein, Allen Atwell, and Richard Aldcroft. Arlene Sklar-Weinstein took LSD during the mid-1960s under the guidance of a psychologist. As recounted by Masters and Houston in *Psychedelic Art*, during the experience she stared for a time into a fire burning in a fireplace. That image became deeply rooted in her mind, and much of her subsequent art incorporated fire images. Masters and Houston quote her description of her experience with LSD.

> The unbelievably beautiful, strange imagery, the expanded concept of time and life in terms of millennia, not years, and most importantly, the sharpened sense of the multi-dimensional qualities in my character, are products of the LSD experience too powerful not to have found their way into my work.

The new medium of psychedelic art also fostered new techniques for creating images. Richard Aldcroft's *Infinity Machine* created psychedelic images through a random process. The machine was a projector, upon which rotated a cylinder containing design elements floating in liquid. The constantly changing patterns of the swirling elements were projected onto a screen. Other artists created whole environments using films, slide projectors, music, dancers, flashing lights, and sounds such as amplified heartbeats, screams, and laughs.

These artists turned discotheques into psychedelic circuses using colored lights that streamed by on walls and ceilings, or blinked, sometimes in attempted synchrony with the music. Artists Jackie Cassen and Rudi Stern contributed to the decorative environment of New York's Cheetah discotheque; Earl Reiback's work swept over parts of the inside of the Electric Circus.

Despite the excitement generated by this new art form, and the drugs that gave artists new insights into their own consciousness, artists were seldom able to work well with their hands while undergoing the psychedelic experience. Those who were able to put their experiences to good use conceived or perceived what they would only later express in their work. As an article in *Psychedelic Review* pointed out at the time, the drug may do no more than provide an experience, and thereafter "the person must himself work with this enlarged frame of reference, this creative schema."

To Be or Not to Be

The minds, eyes, and hands of artists continue to reflect the drug experience. One contemporary artist, Fritz Eichenberg, has updated the medieval theme of the dance-of-death discussed in the chapter "Drugs and Dance." One of these dance

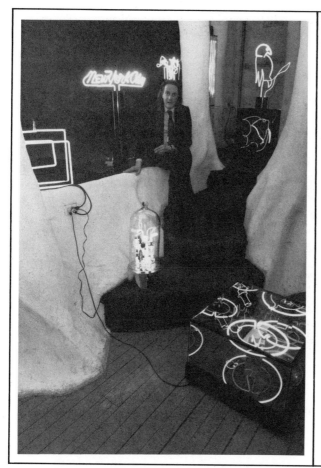

Rudi Stern in his studio. Whereas some psychedelic artists used their drug experiences to enrich their own work, others tried to recreate those experiences for audiences by using blinking lights and other techniques that would recreate distorted modes of perception.

of death wood engravings done by Eichenberg was *Last Cocktail*, which shows a raucous gathering of men and women drinking and getting drunk. Eichenberg wrote:

> A bloody Mary or a Mickey Finn,
> a reefer or some coke—
> it blurs the pain of existential living.
> What if it's temporary? So is life.
> "I'm smashed—I'm stoned—I'm tight—
> my shrink says—oops, I'm sorry—
> What fun! See you, maybe, tomorrow!"

Another Eichenberg engraving, *The Last Shot*, portrays several people lounging around an apartment strewn with beer cans. A couple lying together on the floor are being

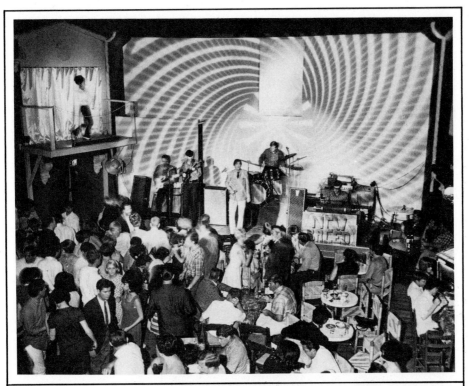

A 1967 crowd enjoys the psychedelic environment of a Dallas nightclub. Since the social upheavals of the 1960s, the abuse of psychedelic drugs has reached far beyond the private domain of artistic creation.

approached by a rat. A young man sitting on a chair is about to receive an injection. The figure holding the needle poised over the man's vein is the figure of death. The accompanying poem reads:

> Yes, Man, I know
> the dice are loaded!
> So what?
> Life is a gamble anyhow!
> You have a choice
> to be or not to be,
> to shoot, snort, smoke
> for kicks or nightmares,
> for heaven or for hell.
> Who cares!
> Who cares?

Eichenberg's updated version of the dance of death stands in sharp contrast to the celebratory moods of the paintings depicting the ancient Dionysian rites. The artists portraying those joyous rituals were paying homage to a popular god whose wine and revelry promised a welcome respite from the drudgery of everyday life. Eichenberg, on the other hand, portrays modern revelers abusing alcohol and other drugs in a self-destructive flight from reality.

These contrasting images illustrate more than what they show. They depict the differing views that different societies have held toward the use of drugs — depending on whether those drugs played important artistic, social, or religious roles, or were tools of self-destruction and social decay.

APPENDIX

State Agencies
for the Prevention and Treatment
of Drug Abuse

ALABAMA
Department of Mental Health
Division of Mental Illness and
  Substance Abuse Community
  Programs
200 Interstate Park Drive
P.O. Box 3710
Montgomery, AL 36193
(205) 271-9253

ALASKA
Department of Health and Social
  Services
Office of Alcoholism and Drug
  Abuse
Pouch H-05-F
Juneau, AK 99811
(907) 586-6201

ARIZONA
Department of Health Services
Division of Behavioral Health
  Services
Bureau of Community Services
Alcohol Abuse and Alcoholism
  Section
2500 East Van Buren
Phoenix, AZ 85008
(602) 255-1238

Department of Health Services
Division of Behavioral Health
  Services
Bureau of Community Services
Drug Abuse Section
2500 East Van Buren
Phoenix, AZ 85008
(602) 255-1240

ARKANSAS
Department of Human Services
Office of Alcohol and Drug Abuse
  Prevention
1515 West 7th Avenue
Suite 310
Little Rock, AR 72202
(501) 371-2603

CALIFORNIA
Department of Alcohol and Drug
  Abuse
111 Capitol Mall
Sacramento, CA 95814
(916) 445-1940

COLORADO
Department of Health
Alcohol and Drug Abuse Division
4210 East 11th Avenue
Denver, CO 80220
(303) 320-6137

CONNECTICUT
Alcohol and Drug Abuse
  Commission
999 Asylum Avenue
3rd Floor
Hartford, CT 06105
(203) 566-4145

DELAWARE
Division of Mental Health
Bureau of Alcoholism and Drug
  Abuse
1901 North Dupont Highway
Newcastle, DE 19720
(302) 421-6101

DISTRICT OF COLUMBIA
Department of Human Services
Office of Health Planning and
  Development
601 Indiana Avenue, NW
Suite 500
Washington, D.C. 20004
(202) 724-5641

FLORIDA
Department of Health and
  Rehabilitative Services
Alcoholic Rehabilitation Program
1317 Winewood Boulevard
Room 187A
Tallahassee, FL 32301
(904) 488-0396

Department of Health and
  Rehabilitative Services
Drug Abuse Program
1317 Winewood Boulevard
Building 6, Room 155
Tallahassee, FL 32301
(904) 488-0900

GEORGIA
Department of Human Resources
Division of Mental Health and
  Mental Retardation
Alcohol and Drug Section
618 Ponce De Leon Avenue, NE
Atlanta, GA 30365-2101
(404) 894-4785

HAWAII
Department of Health
Mental Health Division
Alcohol and Drug Abuse Branch
1250 Punch Bowl Street
P.O. Box 3378
Honolulu, HI 96801
(808) 548-4280

IDAHO
Department of Health and Welfare
Bureau of Preventive Medicine
Substance Abuse Section
450 West State
Boise, ID 83720
(208) 334-4368

ILLINOIS
Department of Mental Health and
  Developmental Disabilities
Division of Alcoholism
160 North La Salle Street
Room 1500
Chicago, IL 60601
(312) 793-2907

Illinois Dangerous Drugs
  Commission
300 North State Street
Suite 1500
Chicago, IL 60610
(312) 822-9860

INDIANA
Department of Mental Health
Division of Addiction Services
429 North Pennsylvania Street
Indianapolis, IN 46204
(317) 232-7816

IOWA
Department of Substance Abuse
505 5th Avenue
Insurance Exchange Building
Suite 202
Des Moines, IA 50319
(515) 281-3641

KANSAS
Department of Social Rehabilitation
Alcohol and Drug Abuse Services
2700 West 6th Street
Biddle Building
Topeka, KS 66606
(913) 296-3925

KENTUCKY
Cabinet for Human Resources
Department of Health Services
Substance Abuse Branch
275 East Main Street
Frankfort, KY 40601
(502) 564-2880

LOUISIANA
Department of Health and Human
  Resources
Office of Mental Health and
  Substance Abuse
655 North 5th Street
P.O. Box 4049
Baton Rouge, LA 70821
(504) 342-2565

MAINE
Department of Human Services
Office of Alcoholism and Drug
  Abuse Prevention
Bureau of Rehabilitation
32 Winthrop Street
Augusta, ME 04330
(207) 289-2781

MARYLAND
Alcoholism Control Administration
201 West Preston Street
Fourth Floor
Baltimore, MD 21201
(301) 383-2977

State Health Department
Drug Abuse Administration
201 West Preston Street
Baltimore, MD 21201
(301) 383-3312

MASSACHUSETTS
Department of Public Health
Division of Alcoholism
755 Boylston Street
Sixth Floor
Boston, MA 02116
(617) 727-1960

Department of Public Health
Division of Drug Rehabilitation
600 Washington Street
Boston, MA 02114
(617) 727-8617

MICHIGAN
Department of Public Health
Office of Substance Abuse Services
3500 North Logan Street
P.O. Box 30035
Lansing, MI 48909
(517) 373-8603

MINNESOTA
Department of Public Welfare
Chemical Dependency Program
  Division
Centennial Building
658 Cedar Street
4th Floor
Saint Paul, MN 55155
(612) 296-4614

MISSISSIPPI
Department of Mental Health
Division of Alcohol and Drug Abuse
1102 Robert E. Lee Building
Jackson, MS 39201
(601) 359-1297

MISSOURI
Department of Mental Health
Division of Alcoholism and Drug
  Abuse
2002 Missouri Boulevard
P.O. Box 687
Jefferson City, MO 65102
(314) 751-4942

MONTANA
Department of Institutions
Alcohol and Drug Abuse Division
1539 11th Avenue
Helena, MT 59620
(406) 449-2827

NEBRASKA
Department of Public Institutions
Division of Alcoholism and Drug
Abuse
801 West Van Dorn Street
P.O. Box 94728
Lincoln, NB 68509
(402) 471-2851, Ext. 415

NEVADA
Department of Human Resources
Bureau of Alcohol and Drug Abuse
505 East King Street
Carson City, NV 89710
(702) 885-4790

NEW HAMPSHIRE
Department of Health and Welfare
Office of Alcohol and Drug Abuse
    Prevention
Hazen Drive
Health and Welfare Building
Concord, NH 03301
(603) 271-4627

NEW JERSEY
Department of Health
Division of Alcoholism
129 East Hanover Street CN 362
Trenton, NJ 08625
(609) 292-8949

Department of Health
Division of Narcotic and Drug
    Abuse Control
129 East Hanover Street CN 362
Trenton, NJ 08625
(609) 292-8949

NEW MEXICO
Health and Environment Department
Behavioral Services Division
Substance Abuse Bureau
725 Saint Michaels Drive
P.O. Box 968
Santa Fe, NM 87503
(505) 984-0020, Ext. 304

NEW YORK
Division of Alcoholism and Alcohol
    Abuse
194 Washington Avenue
Albany, NY 12210
(518) 474-5417

Division of Substance Abuse
    Services
Executive Park South
Box 8200
Albany, NY 12203
(518) 457-7629

NORTH CAROLINA
Department of Human Resources
Division of Mental Health, Mental
    Retardation and Substance Abuse
    Services
Alcohol and Drug Abuse Services
325 North Salisbury Street
Albemarle Building
Raleigh, NC 27611
(919) 733-4670

NORTH DAKOTA
Department of Human Services
Division of Alcoholism and Drug
    Abuse
State Capitol Building
Bismarck, ND 58505
(701) 224-2767

OHIO
Department of Health
Division of Alcoholism
246 North High Street
P.O. Box 118
Columbus, OH 43216
(614) 466-3543

Department of Mental Health
Bureau of Drug Abuse
65 South Front Street
Columbus, OH 43215
(614) 466-9023

OKLAHOMA
Department of Mental Health
Alcohol and Drug Programs
4545 North Lincoln Boulevard
Suite 100 East Terrace
P.O. Box 53277
Oklahoma City, OK 73152
(405) 521-0044

OREGON
Department of Human Resources
Mental Health Division
Office of Programs for Alcohol and
  Drug Problems
2575 Bittern Street, NE
Salem, OR 97310
(503) 378-2163

PENNSYLVANIA
Department of Health
Office of Drug and Alcohol
  Programs
Commonwealth and Forster Avenues
Health and Welfare Building
P.O. Box 90
Harrisburg, PA 17108
(717) 787-9857

RHODE ISLAND
Department of Mental Health,
  Mental Retardation and Hospitals
Division of Substance Abuse
Substance Abuse Administration
  Building
Cranston, RI 02920
(401) 464-2091

SOUTH CAROLINA
Commission on Alcohol and Drug
  Abuse
3700 Forest Drive
Columbia, SC 29204
(803) 758-2521

SOUTH DAKOTA
Department of Health
Division of Alcohol and Drug Abuse
523 East Capitol, Joe Foss Building
Pierre, SD 57501
(605) 773-4806

TENNESSEE
Department of Mental Health and
  Mental Retardation
Alcohol and Drug Abuse Services
505 Deaderick Street
James K. Polk Building,
  Fourth Floor
Nashville, TN 37219
(615) 741-1921

TEXAS
Commission on Alcoholism
809 Sam Houston State Office
  Building
Austin, TX 78701
(512) 475-2577
Department of Community Affairs
Drug Abuse Prevention Division
2015 South Interstate Highway 35
P.O. Box 13166
Austin, TX 78711
(512) 443-4100

UTAH
Department of Social Services
Division of Alcoholism and Drugs
150 West North Temple
Suite 350
P.O. Box 2500
Salt Lake City, UT 84110
(801) 533-6532

VERMONT
Agency of Human Services
Department of Social and
  Rehabilitation Services
Alcohol and Drug Abuse Division
103 South Main Street
Waterbury, VT 05676
(802) 241-2170

VIRGINIA
Department of Mental Health and
  Mental Retardation
Division of Substance Abuse
109 Governor Street
P.O. Box 1797
Richmond, VA 23214
(804) 786-5313

WASHINGTON
Department of Social and Health
  Service
Bureau of Alcohol and Substance
  Abuse
Office Building—44 W
Olympia, WA 98504
(206) 753-5866

WEST VIRGINIA
Department of Health
Office of Behavioral Health Services
Division on Alcoholism and Drug
  Abuse
1800 Washington Street East
Building 3 Room 451
Charleston, WV 25305
(304) 348-2276

WISCONSIN
Department of Health and Social
  Services
Division of Community Services
Bureau of Community Programs
Alcohol and Other Drug Abuse
  Program Office
1 West Wilson Street
P.O. Box 7851
Madison, WI 53707
(608) 266-2717

WYOMING
Alcohol and Drug Abuse Programs
Hathaway Building
Cheyenne, WY 82002
(307) 777-7115, Ext. 7118

GUAM
Mental Health & Substance Abuse
  Agency
P.O. Box 20999
Guam 96921

PUERTO RICO
Department of Addiction Control
  Services
Alcohol Abuse Programs
P.O. Box B-Y Rio Piedras Station
Rio Piedras, PR 00928
(809) 763-5014

Department of Addiction Control
  Services
Drug Abuse Programs
P.O. Box B-Y Rio Piedras Station
Rio Piedras, PR 00928
(809) 764-8140

VIRGIN ISLANDS
Division of Mental Health,
  Alcoholism & Drug Dependency
  Services
P.O. Box 7329
Saint Thomas, Virgin Islands 00801
(809) 774-7265

AMERICAN SAMOA
LBJ Tropical Medical Center
Department of Mental Health Clinic
Pago Pago, American Samoa 96799

TRUST TERRITORIES
Director of Health Services
Office of the High Commissioner
Saipan, Trust Territories 96950

Further Reading

Abel, Ernest L. *Marijuana: The First Twelve Thousand Years*. New York: McGraw Hill, 1982.

Brownlow, Kevin. *Hollywood: The Pioneers*. New York: Alfred A. Knopf, 1979.

Hayter, Alethea. *Opium and the Romantic Imagination*. Berkeley and Los Angeles: University of California Press, 1968.

Pareles, Jon, and Romanowski, Patricia, eds. *The Rolling Stone Encyclopedia of Rock & Roll*. New York: Rolling Stone Press/ Summit Books, 1983.

Tytell, John. *Naked Angels: The Lives and Literature of the Beat Generation*. New York: McGraw Hill, 1976.

Whitcomb, Ian. *After the Ball: Pop Music from Rag to Rock*. New York: Simon and Schuster, 1972.

Glossary

absinthe a green, toxic liqueur made from a combination of brandy, wormwood, and other herbs

abstain to refrain deliberately and often from an action or practice

addiction a condition caused by repeated drug use, characterized by a compulsive urge to continue using the drug, a tendency to increase the dosage, and physiological and/or psychological dependence

alkaloid one of many organic substances that contain nitrogen and strongly affect body functions; drugs such as morphine and cocaine are alkaloids

amphetamine a drug that stimulates the nervous system; generally used as a mood elevator, energizer, antidepressant, and appetite depressant

bacchante a riotous or frenzied woman. The term is often associated with followers of the Greek god Dionysus who would gather to participate in orgiastic rites of worship. Also called a maenad

beatniks people in the 1960s who expressed a nonconformist social philosophy by the unconventional way they dressed and behaved

bootlegging the act of smuggling or selling illegally, often associated with the illegal sale of liquor

cormorant a large, black bird associated with the sea

counterculture the lifestyle of people who reject accepted norms of social behavior and/or established values

cubism a school of art in which objects are represented as various geometric shapes

danse macabre French term for the macabre dance or dance of death that originated in the Middle Ages following a scourge of plagues in Europe. The dance consisted of a procession symbolically following a death figure, often to the grave itself

demonologist a person who studies and believes in demons (devils or evil spirits)

diptych a painting consisting of two panels hinged together and often illustrating multiple scenes

dithyramb a hymn to the god Dionysus in ancient Greece

freebasing a potent and dangerous method whereby street cocaine is mixed with ammonium hydroxide and heated, then smoked in a pipe for a quick and addictive high

hashish the leaves and soft portions of the hemp plant, which are dried and either chewed or smoked for their narcotic effects

hyperesthesia increased sensitivity of the sensory organs

impressionism a late 19th-century school of painting that worked with the dynamics of light to represent objects

laudanum an alcoholic extract of opium used for sedative purposes

lithograph a picture made as a result of a printing process called lithography, in which ink adheres to parts of a treated surface featuring a design rather than to the entire surface area

mandala in Oriental art, a circular, concentric arrangement of shapes representing the cosmos

morality play a type of drama popular in the 16th century that taught moral lessons and featured characters representing the values or qualities that man believed in

narcotic a drug that produces sleep and pain relief pain in small doses, but stupors and unconsciousness in larger amounts; examples of these drugs are opium, codeine, morphine and heroin

opium a hallucinogenic drug made from the milky juice of the poppy plant *Papaver somniferum* that is chewed, smoked or used for sedative purposes in medicine

orgiastic a state of indulging to the point of wild revelry

peyote a hallucinogenic drug prepared from a Mexican cactus plant of this same name

physical dependence adaption of the body to the presence of a drug such that its absence produces withdrawal symptoms

pop art a style of art that often deals with images portrayed in posters and comic strips

prohibition era a period dating from 1920 to 1933 when the production and sale of liquor was illegal in the United States

protagonist the leading character in a work of literature

psilocin an unstable ingredient related to the neurotransmitter serotonin that is found in *Psilocybe*, a genus of psychoactive mushrooms

psilocybin an acidic phosphoric acid ester related to serotonin and a psychoactive ingredient in *Psilocybe*

psychedelic producing hallucinations or having mind-altering or mind-expanding properties

psychological dependence a condition in which the drug user craves a drug to maintain a sense of well-being and feels discomfort when deprived of it

Puritan a member of the 16th- and 17th-century English Protestant group that advocated simpler forms of church ceremony as well as strictness in morals and behavior

realism the representation of objects in a form that is true to nature

Renaissance a period from the 14th to 16th centuries marked by a reawakening of arts and literature in Europe

romanticism a literary or artistic style in which passion and extremes of grandeur or beauty define the object as opposed to a portrayal marked by exact proportions

seer a prophet or someone who sees visions

shaman a priest or witch doctor found in various cultures who claims to have sole contact with the gods and the power to make contact with them

Shiite a member of the Shiah sect, one of the two branches of Islam. Shiites believe Ali is the first successor of Muhammad

soporific a substance that causes sleep

Sufi a member of the mystical Muslim sect who leads a starkly simple life for religious purposes

surrealism a movement in 20th century art and literature that attempts to represent what is in the subconscious by depicting dreamlike objects and events

temperance self-restraint or abstinence from drinking alcoholic beverages

tolerance a decrease of susceptibility to the effects of a drug due to its continued administration, resulting in the user's need to increase the drug dosage in order to achieve desired effects

withdrawal the physiological and psychological effects of discontinued use of a drug

Picture Credits

Art Resource: pp. 12, 20, 32, 90, 91, 92, 98; The Bettmann Archive: pp. 8, 10, 24, 28, 30, 33, 36, 39, 40, 41, 42, 43, 46, 48, 50, 54, 61, 66, 69, 73, 74, 80, 81, 82, 88; Bildarchiv Foto Marburg/Art Resource: pp. 95, 99; Bridgeman/ Art Resource: p. 94; Ann Charters: p. 56; Giraudon/Art Resource: p. 96; The Metropolitan Museum of Art: p. 26; Paramount Pictures: pp. 72, 77; Arthur Sirdofsky/Art Resource: p. 18; SNARK/Art Resource: pp. 22, 37, 55, 85; UPI/ Bettmann Newsphotos: pp. 52, 67, 78, 86, 103, 105, 106; Warner Bros.: pp. 64, 71

Index

Marc Kusinitz, Ph.D., is a science writer currently working freelance for *New Medical Science,* a bimonthly publication distributed to physicians. In addition to having served as news editor for the *New York State Journal of Medicine* and associate editor for *Scholastic Science World,* Dr. Kusinitz has written articles for *Science Digest* and *The New York Times.*

Solomon H. Snyder, M.D., is Distinguished Service Professor of Neuroscience, Pharmacology and Psychiatry at The Johns Hopkins University School of Medicine. He has served as president of the Society for Neuroscience and in 1978 received the Albert Lasker Award in Medical Research. He has authored *Uses of Marijuana, Madness and the Brain, The Troubled Mind, Biological Aspects of Mental Disorder,* and edited *Perspective in Neuropharmacology: A Tribute to Julius Axelrod.* Professor Snyder was a research associate with Dr. Axelrod at the National Institutes of Health.

Barry L. Jacobs, Ph.D., is currently a professor in the program of neuroscience at Princeton University. Professor Jacobs is author of *Serotonin Neurotransmission and Behavior* and *Hallucinogens: Neurochemical, Behavioral and Clinical Perspectives.* He has written many journal articles in the field of neuroscience and contributed numerous chapters to books on behavior and brain science. He has been a member of several panels of the National Institute of Mental Health.

Joann Ellison Rodgers, M.S. (Columbia), became Deputy Director of Public Affairs and Director of Media Relations for the Johns Hopkins Medical Institutions in Baltimore, Maryland, in 1984 after 18 years as an award-winning science journalist and widely read columnist for the Hearst newspapers.